KNOWLEDGE FOR HEALTH CARE PRACTICE

A Guide to Using Research Evidence

Sarah Jo Brown, PhD, RN
Principal and Consultant
Practice-Research Integrations
Norwich, Vermont

D1516485

W.B. SAUNDERS COMPANY
A Division of Harcourt Brace & Company
Philadelphia   London   Toronto   Montreal   Sydney   Tokyo

W.B. SAUNDERS COMPANY

A Division of Harcourt Brace & Company

The Curtis Center
Independence Square West
Philadelphia, Pennsylvania 19106

Library of Congress Cataloging-in-Publication Data

Brown, Sarah Jo
Knowledge for health care practice : a guide to using research
evidence / Sarah Jo Brown.—1st ed.

p.   cm.

Includes bibliographical references.

ISBN 0–7216–7803–3

1. Evidence-based medicine—Handbooks, manuals, etc.
  2. Medicine—Research—Evaluation—Handbooks, manuals, etc.
  3. Medical care—Decision making—Handbooks, manuals, etc.   I. Title.

R853.R46 B76   1999

610'.72—dc21   98–27551

KNOWLEDGE FOR HEALTH CARE PRACTICE:
A Guide to Using Research Evidence   ISBN 0–7216–7803–3

Printed in the United States of America.

Last digit is the print number: 9   8   7   6   5   4   3   2   1

CONTRIBUTOR

Fred Pond, BA, MLS

Nursing Library Services Coordinator,
Matthews-Fuller Health Sciences Library,
Biomedical Libraries,
Dartmouth-Hitchcock Medical Center,
Lebanon, New Hampshire

Searching for Studies

Preface

As we approach the 21st century, all health care disciplines are faced with large bodies of research findings. The public and the health care professions expect that practitioners will use research findings as a source of knowledge in treating individual patients and in designing care for populations of patients. Yet the practitioner who seeks to incorporate research findings into practice soon realizes that locating, appraising, and deciding whether to use research evidence is a complex and time-consuming endeavor. Moreover, specific advice regarding how to do it is thin and fractured.

Filling some gaps

General guidance regarding the overall process of using research in practice exists, as does detailed advice about how to critique and appraise individual studies. However, there is a gap between these two forms of guidance: specific advice regarding how to appraise the collective evidence from two or more studies is lacking. Meta-analysis is, of course, one such method, but others need to be developed and specifically described. The ideas presented in Chapter 9 represent a beginning endeavor at developing strategies and methods that can be used by practitioners who encounter several studies on a particular topic. Thus, the ideas offered in this book attempt to fill some of the gaps in the literature on research utilization.

There are three main tasks facing the practitioner who reads research findings with the intent of possibly changing practice. She or he must: appraise the scientific credibility of the findings, appraise the clinical significance of the findings, and decide whether the findings would be likely to hold up within a particular population and setting. Although it would seem that research textbooks should be helpful in learning how to go about performing these tasks, they are often disappointing. The fact is that most research texts are written from the perspective of how to conduct research, and even though they may have the word *utilization* in their title or several chapters on research utilization, the specific activities required to prudently incorporate research into practice receive little attention.

An additional issue is that the array of research evidence practitioners encounter during their professional reading is quite broad. Reporting of research findings takes many forms, including reports of single studies, meta-analyses, integrative research review, and research-based practice guidelines. The studies reported have been conducted using a variety of research designs (some quite complex), and findings are reported using a miscellany of measures, statistics, and portrayals. Not uncommonly, several or many studies may have been conducted on a topic, each with slightly (or greatly) different findings. The approach of this book recognizes all this diversity rather than glossing over it.

Three pathways of research-based practice are recognized: one for evidence in the form of state-of-the science summaries, another for collective evidence from two or more studies, and a third for single studies (when only one study on a topic is available). Specific sets of appraisal questions are provided for five different study designs, and sets of questions for the appraisal of collective evidence regarding four general categories of clinical topics are set forth. Although this approach requires the practitioner to think clearly about a clinical question and about the type of research evidence being considered, once this has been done the guidance provided is specific and highly relevant to the particular form of research evidence and to the clinical topic.

The guidance provided takes the forms of pathways, steps, and specific questions to guide you through the process of appraising research evidence; in that sense it truly is a handbook but it is not a cookbook. You will need to do much more than just follow the recommended sequence of activities and answer the questions superficially. Concentration will be required to grasp the more difficult sections, you may need to supplement your reading by referring to a research text, and the decisions you will be asked to make about the research evidence and about whether you should use it in your practice will require thinking that is both analytical and reflective.

Perhaps the advice Sophie received from her mysterious mentor who was showing her around the world of philosophic literature applies to the use of this book also:

> "Thank you for your attention, Sophie. It is not unlikely that you will need to read this chapter two or three times before you understand it all. But understanding will always require some effort. You probably wouldn't admire a friend who was good at everything if it cost her no effort." (Gaarder, 1994).

Who might want to use this book

This book is written for heath care practitioners and students in professional educational programs; the examples used are from many health care disciplines and clinical specialties. Multidisciplinary clinical groups and small group practices who are committed to making their practice more research-based will find the book useful, as will members of a hospital research committee or a multidisciplinary group who are planning a new clinical program or designing a clinical path. Several suggestions are made in Chapter 3 regarding how a multidisciplinary group might organize itself. The individual practitioner who wants to learn more about how to read and appraise research reports and summaries would receive step-by-step guidance in research-based practice.

Of note is the strong suggestion that *basic* knowledge of statistics, research designs, types of data, and principles of data analysis is required to fully benefit from this book. Although this knowledge can be acquired as you proceed if you take the time to branch off and acquire the required knowledge for each chapter and section from a research text.

Although in professional health care eduction the book could be useful at several levels, students in post baccalaureate clinical programs would probably get the most from it. However, the author has actually used the book in a first research course for RN-to-BSN students who already had a basic statistics course. It was a rigorous course; they had to learn both basic research methodology content and appraisal of research evidence in one semester—still, the students reported learning a great deal and said it was worth the effort they put into it.

Learning strategies

The recommended use of the book would be in a two-semester course focused on research-based practice. Research methodology content required to be a consumer of research and the research-based practice content of this book could be taught in a highly integrated manner. The integration could be developed around either clinical questions or types of studies and the different forms of research evidence (single studies, collective evidence, and state-of-the science summaries).

Alternatively, this book and a research text could be used as the major resources made available to students in a research-based practice course taught using problem-based learning. Students would be asked to identify a clinical problem for which they need research evidence, and by following the appropriate pathway presented in this book they would be guided through an experience in using research evidence to answer a particular clinical problem. They would read specific research methodology content as needed to understand and appraise certain evidence; if they were required to answer two or three clinical problems in this way they would be exposed to quite a bit of research methodology content and most of the content of this book during the course.

Maximal learning will occur if the reader is an active learner. Starting in Chapter 4, the active learner would identify a clinical question or topic of interest, proceed to search for and retrieve relevant evidence, and then perform the activities that compose each of the appraisal pathways. Actual use of at least one set of questions from Chapters 8, 9, and 10 provides practice in database searching and discriminating between types of evidence, as well as an opportunity to experience the logic of appraisal for that type of evidence. Examples of appraisals for each pathway are included in the appendix, but they do not replace the reader actually using the questions provided to appraise a specific form of evidence.

Work-in-progress

Considerable very useful work regarding the incorporation of various forms of research evidence into practice has already been done by others—the work presented in this book has built upon those prior contributions. However, much work still remains to be done to further develop and refine the analytical and synthesis tools required to appraise the worthiness and readiness of research findings for use in practice. These tools are needed by practitioners who seek to fully utilize the wealth of research evidence available to improve patient care and patient outcomes. The initiatives of the Agency for Health Care Policy and Research of the U.S. Department of Health and Human Services and of other evidence-based centers in other countries to establish evidence-based centers for the purpose of producing evidence reports will certainly advance the development of such tools, as well as make evidence summaries available to practitioners. These initiatives, however, will not completely relieve the individual practitioner of the responsibility of being able to read and appraise research evidence to answer questions that arise in his or her practice.

SARAH JO BROWN

Gaarder, J. (1994). *Sophie's world: A novel about the history of philosophy.* (P. Moller, Trans.) New York: Berkley.

Acknowledgments

An author has ideas but relies on others to provide encouragement when confidence is flagging, honest critique when confidence is soaring, alternative thinking when dealing with difficult content, and tea breaks when absorption in writing is excessive. Chris Senger put up with me during the writing of this book. Ethie Slate worked with me line-by-line, chapter-by-chapter to produce coherency and clarity of thought. The Norwich University RN-to-BSN students in the Upper Valley Cohort (Class of '98) worked with an early version of the book, made helpful suggestions, and assured me that the approach was useful to practitioners. Fred Pond, the Nursing Librarian at the Dartmouth-Hitchcock Medical Center, contributed the chapter on searching for studies; the content was difficult to cull and organize—I just could not have written that chapter as well. Lastly, many unknown reviewers thoughtfully read the manuscript during the proposal stage and during the final editing stage; I read and re-read their reactions and suggestions and made changes based on them. To all these friends and colleagues, I express deeply felt gratitude.

sjb

Contents

1

Clinical Knowledge

All health care practitioners use certain treatments, therapies, interventions, and approaches over and over again, and seldom stop to think about how they came to have confidence in them. The original source may have been a textbook, journal article, respected colleague, professor, or continuing education speaker. Although practice knowledge inevitably is a collage put together from many different sources, in order for care to be soundly based and contemporary, research-based knowledge must contribute to that collage.

The collage of clinical knowledge used by a practitioner is composed of information, insights, and maxims derived from diverse personal and professional sources (Box 1–1). Knowledge produced by research has the virtue of having been systematically developed and tested; still, the range of conditions under which the findings will hold often is not known. Thus, knowledge produced by research is dependable in the general sense, but the practitioner must use discretion in deciding whether and how to use research findings in practice. Care actions and decisions based on trial and error, acquired insights, intuitive responses, and interpersonal impressions have been called "experience-based care" because the practitioner relies on past experience and personal interpretation to sort out and make sense of what is being said, seen, and sensed during a clinical encounter. It follows, then, that care based on logical thinking and reasoning could be called "reasoning-based care." This rationale for care is used when a practitioner uses knowledge from physiology, pathophysiology, pharmacology, or behavioral science to understand what is going on in a situation. Another rationale for care is authority. When a practitioner uses a care modality because it was recommended in a reference book, in a report from experts, or by a trusted colleague, the care could be called "authority-based care."

The newest source of knowledge for practice, quality data, comes from what has been called improvement science which includes all the methods and knowledge being produced by continuous quality improvement projects to evaluate and improve clinical care within health care agencies and

Box 1–1
Clinical Knowledge Sources

- Research
- Experience
- Reasoning
- Authority
- Quality data
- Patient's account

systems. Although the methods are not completely scientific in the traditional sense, they do involve problem identification, systematic data collection, standards-based analysis, and findings-based decisions. Unlike traditional science, which aims to produce knowledge that can be generalized across settings, quality improvement monitoring and evaluation produce knowledge that serves the purpose of improving patient care and patient outcomes at the single agency or health care system level. This knowledge should be recognized as a form of evidence that can and does influence individual and agency clinical practice.

All these sources of professional knowledge inform clinical decision making, and no one of them can, or should, serve without the support of the others. Moreover, even though in theory these sources of professional knowledge can be delineated, in practice they are fused with one another. What started out as research-based knowledge gets modified by experience, or the practitioner blends experience-based knowledge with authority-based knowledge to evolve a way of treating a particular problem based on the types of patients she sees. These forms of professional knowledge must, of course, be combined with the patient's knowledge. To fully and accurately understand what is going on and to make helpful and acceptable recommendations, the patient's account of his experiences, his view of his situation, and his expectations and preferences must be taken into account.

This book focuses solely on using research findings as a source of knowledge to shape and design one's practice. The advocacy of research-based practice inherent in this book rests on the assumption that the methods of science produce dependable and useful forms of knowledge about health, illness, and health care that are useful across clinical situations. Nevertheless, a case for research evidence as the supreme form of evidence will not be offered because this would diminish the other sources. Humanistic health care has always used knowledge from diverse sources; it has always been a blend of art and science. Experience, logic, intuition, local conditions and values, and creativity must co-mingle with the contributions of science to produce humane, effective health care.

RESEARCH-BASED PRACTICE

Recently there has been a renewed call in the health care professions to base care on the best research evidence available. The terms "research-based practice" and "evidence-based health care" have been used to refer to the critical appraisal of research findings and the decisions regarding whether and how to use the findings in the care of patients. Broad application of these terms recognizes that in addition to using research findings to guide management and treatment actions, practitioners also seek knowledge produced by research to help them understand patients' and families' experiences with health and illness. Research findings can enrich practitioners' understanding of how illness affects the lives of patients and their families; they can direct attention to the psychological and social factors that influence a person's health-related behaviors and responses; and they can provide descriptions of interpersonal approaches and actions that make the caregiving relationship more comfortable for patients.

The following definition of research-based practice was developed to recognize: (a) the direct and the subtle influences of research on practitioners' thinking and actions, (b) the influence of findings from individual studies as well as the collective evidence from two or more studies, and (c) the critical appraisal aspect of research-based practice.

Research-based practice is health care practitioners' considered use of research findings and collective research evidence to shape general approaches to care, specific courses of action, and recommendations made to individual patients.

Research-based practice is not an absolute way of practicing, because almost every clinical encounter requires a practitioner to address an array of issues and to choose among several approaches; for some of these issues substantial research evidence may exist, whereas for others the evidence may be scant or nonexistent. Even when research findings exist, practitioners must still decide if and how the findings should influence the care of individual patients. For these reasons, research-based practice is a relative way of practicing, a way in which the practitioner makes an effort to integrate research findings into clinical thinking and decision making while recognizing that effective health care practice is more than the mere application of scientific knowledge.

REASONS FOR ENGAGING IN RESEARCH-BASED PRACTICE

Much of clinical health research is conducted for the purpose of producing knowledge needed to assist patients in achieving positive health outcomes. Use of that knowledge toward the goals of better patient outcomes clearly is the main reason why practitioners make the considerable effort required to engage in research-based practice. However, patients also benefit indirectly from research-based practice as it enhances professional discourse and contributes to the intellectual challenge and satisfaction professionals experience in their work. Engaging in research-based practice is timely because a great deal of health care research is being conducted and can be easily and quickly located using electronic database searching media.

Increased Availability of and Accessibility to Research Reports

In contrast with the not-too-distant past, when you look for studies on a specific health care topic it is highly likely that some will have been done.

There are more randomized clinical trials, more studies describing patients' experiences with health and illness, and more studies describing the factors that influence how individuals and families respond to troubling health states. This diversity of topics on which research has been done provides a rich source of information for all health care providers.

Health care research is also more relevant to the realities of practice in ways that it was not in the past. As recently as five years ago, the cost of care was not included as a variable in most clinical intervention studies. Now the situation is quite different. The number of studies examining cost-related factors, such as hospital admission rates and use of expensive health re-sources, and the number of studies examining delivery issues, such as referral patterns and barriers to care, are remarkable. The cost and acceptability of a modality are clearly determinants of whether it will be adopted in the modern health care marketplace; increasingly, there is a growing amount of research-based data about these issues as they relate to the clinical effective-ness of various options.

The accessibility of research finding has been improved by the inclusion of research reports in clinical specialty journals, not just in research journals as in the past. The increased number of state-of-the-science summaries being published in clinical journals enables practitioners to learn about many studies that have been done on a topic by reading just one article. Perhaps the best-known summaries are provided by the Agency for Health Care Research & Policy (AHCPR) on 17 common health care conditions, includ-ing pressure ulcers in adults, cataracts in adults, otitis media in young children, smoking cessation, and urinary incontinence. These guidelines consist of systematic reviews of relevant studies and specific clinical guide-lines; the guidelines include Quick Reference Guides for Clinicians and Patient's Guides. Several other sources are producing high-quality state-of-the-science summaries and research-based clinical guidelines (described in Chapter 10).

State-of-the-science summaries, individual studies, and research-based guidelines can be located by searching computerized health science data-bases using proprietary CD ROM systems, the Internet, and Telnet (which provides access to the holdings catalogues at university and public libraries). Many small hospitals have one of these forms of access to a database, and belong to interlibrary loan networks to assist their staff members in obtaining research reports and other health care literature. All these sources together assure that research reports and summaries of research are, and will be in the future, increasingly accessible to practitioners without the need to travel to distant resources. An extensive discussion of how to access and use many of these resources is provided in Chapter 5.

Refined Criteria for Appraising Findings

In addition to more research and easier access to study reports and state-of-the-science summaries, the strategies for systematically appraising findings and deciding whether and how to change practice have been refined by several health care disciplines. Since the late 1970s, nurses have published guidelines for critiquing studies and models for using research in clinical practice (Stetler and Marram, 1976), and have conducted research utilization projects (Horsley, Crane, Crabtree, and Wood, 1983). These models and projects made it evident that appraising the findings of a study for use in practice has a very different objective than "critiquing a study," which many health care professionals learned to do during their basic education. The main purpose of learning critiques is to apply the standards for well-conducted studies to evaluating the scientific soundness of particular studies; typically, 20 to 60 questions help identify the methodological strengths and weaknesses of a study. Although this approach is undoubtedly useful for student learning, the practitioner must go beyond evaluating the scientific soundness of a study to also consider the practical significance and applicability of its findings.

More recently, physicians have developed detailed methods for appraising the validity of research findings and answering the question of whether the results of a study will help in caring for patients in a particular setting. McMasters University in Canada and the University of Oxford in England were among the first to develop centers for evidence-based medicine, but many others now exist around the world. Both universities maintain sites on the Internet that provide specific guidance for the practitioner seeking to engage in research-based practice, as well for educators who want to incorporate research-based practice into professional health care provider curriculums.

The work of AHCPR in conducting research reviews and publishing clinical practice guidelines, and more recently, their funding of evidence-based practice centers, has also advanced the development of analytical and integrative tools for summarizing research findings. The result of these activities and of the Cochrane Collaboration (Cochrane Library, 1998) has been the publication of more, high-quality summaries of research on a wide variety of topics in and across all health care disciplines.

Persuasive Rationale for Change

Another reason to move toward research-based practice is that research data provide an objective rationale for choosing one approach over another. When differences of opinion arise regarding how to manage a problem, generally the approach with the greatest research support should be tried first. As more research about issues of concern to disciplines other than medicine becomes available, these disciplines are able to use that research to advocate their perspectives and provide rationale for the interventions, therapies, and strategies used by their disciplines. Research findings are a respected rationale for care, and are often persuasive when logic, experience, and personal insight are not honored.

When using research findings to advocate for a certain point of view or course of action, it is important, however, to obtain the full report, read it thoroughly, and appraise the credibility of the findings. Relying on the abstract alone, or extracting the findings without appraising how well the study was done would be a slipshod approach to using the research. It is important to review the study and make a thoughtful appraisal of the findings, for it is possible that the study may have been weakly designed and therefore its findings are not to be trusted. The point of using research to justify a point of view is not to intimidate, but rather to establish that your ideas are more than personal opinion, that they are backed with objective evidence, and that you value research-based information.

It behooves all practitioners to know the research studies and findings pertaining to the group of patients for whom they regularly provide care, and most particularly the studies that pertain to the issues they are responsible for managing. Studies that convey what patients' experiences have been like, what their concerns and preferences are, and what they think has worked for them are also valuable in advocating for certain courses of action. Studies comparing patient outcomes associated with two or more ways of doing something often provide an objective basis for choosing one over the other. Being able to cite research findings puts all professional providers on the same footing, because it neutralizes personal opinion, dominance behaviors, interpersonal assertiveness, and disciplinary value differences. It should be noted, however, that the phrase "research shows . . ." is an overused phrase; to be convincing, one must be able to cite the specifics of studies: authors, journal, site where the study was conducted, profile of the patient sample, methods, and findings. It is also important to be familiar with other studies relevant to the issue, particularly those with findings different from those you are citing.

Professional Satisfaction

Practitioners who set aside time for locating and appraising research relevant to their practice will find that their day-to-day professional life is more interesting and satisfying. The satisfaction comes from acting in a more reflective manner—and less from routine and habit. The regular infusion of new ideas and the more thoughtful way of practicing can only feel more intellectually fulfilling. Then, as you learn to share the research rationale for recommending a certain course of action with patients, the satisfactions that come from helping someone else make informed decisions about his own care can be realized. Finally, being informed about current research provides you with a rich knowledge base to bring to professional conversations and consultations.

WILL MY PATIENTS EXPERIENCE BETTER OUTCOMES?

The ultimate question still must be "If I adopt a research-based action, will the patients I care for experience improved outcomes?" Unfortunately, the answer to this important question is not clear-cut. Although the benefits of research-based practice to patients are logically and intuitively compelling, definitive evidence is lacking. It is logical to expect that methods that have been found to produce "better" patient outcomes in research studies should produce better patient outcomes when incorporated into everyday practice. However, there are three reasons why this may not be so.

Works for Some, Not for Others

First, the conclusion of most intervention studies is that a certain treatment or intervention worked better *on average* than did the treatment received by the control group (Barlow and Hersen, 1984). In essence, this means that the experimental approach was better on average than was the control approach. Although the experimental treatment may have worked well for most people, it may not have worked as well for others, and may not have worked at all for some. Therefore, it is left for the clinician to determine which category a particular client or clients fall into. The clinician who tries a therapy that has been found to be beneficial in well-conducted research is providing high-quality care because there is objective, empirical support for the therapy. Nevertheless, even when relying on research-based approaches, experience will still need to be tapped to decide if a particular patient will benefit, or is benefiting, from it.

Different Conditions

The second reason why research findings may not transfer well into everyday practice is that the controlled conditions of research studies are often not in place in everyday practice, and variations in the way the treatment is delivered may affect the outcomes experienced. The attempt to use research in practice, in a sense, represents a replication of the study from which the findings came. This replication, however, inevitably introduces new setting conditions and often slight variations on how an intervention or therapy is delivered that were not present in the original study. These changes in conditions may lie outside the range of conditions to which the original findings apply.

Profile of the Research Participants

As important, the persons participating in the study may not have been like the patients you see. Thus, you should take into account the profile of the persons who contributed the data, and note differences (or similarities) between them and those you see. If a study was conducted on the ability of urban, working women with rheumatoid arthritis to fulfill their family role responsibilities, the findings may be of limited use to you if you provide care to a population of farming and logging families.

Just because your patients are not like those who participated in the study is not a reason to dismiss the findings. Rather, differences must be recognized as a factor that may limit the extent to which your populations will respond to an illness experience or intervention in the same way those in the study did. The possibility also exists, of course, that the research-based methods may work even better or with more patients than they did under the research conditions.

In summary, the issue of whether your patients would experience better outcomes if you as a provider adopted more research-based methods cannot be answered definitively, but logic and probability predict that better outcomes are more likely, particularly if the patients studied are similar to your patients. In addition, careful attention to the conditions and procedures used in the research study will enable you to more accurately predict how likely the results of a study or group of studies are to transfer to your everyday practice.

RELATED TERMS

The term "research-based practice" will be used throughout this book, rather than "evidence-based practice" or "research utilization," which are other widely used terms. "Research-based practice" was chosen because it specifies research findings as the specific form of evidence being considered as a basis for professional actions and decisions. A focus on research-based knowledge shouldn't isolate the use of research knowledge from the other forms of evidence; rather, it affords research-based knowledge a prominent place in the collage of evidence used in practice.

For many years the term "research utilization" was used to refer to the process by which scientifically produced knowledge is transferred to practice. Embedded in this term is a distinction between two closely related but distinct processes: conducting research and using research—hence, a distinction between the production of knowledge and the utilization of knowledge. Most people have a much clearer understanding of what is meant by conducting research than they do of what is meant by using research. Conducting research is often viewed as a precise, erudite activity, whereas using research is viewed as a mundane, common sense kind of activity. In reality, both activities require knowledge regarding the research process and the ability to think analytically. Using research is a more complex skill than most people realize; it requires knowledge about research methods as well as a disciplined effort to critically appraise research in relation to current practice.

SUMMARY

Engaging in research-based practice involves systematically appraising research evidence and deciding whether to integrate the findings into clinical practice. The use of research findings from a single study or research evidence from two or more studies, however, should not stand apart from the other sources of clinical knowledge that also serve as bases for high-quality, individualized care. It is also important to note that the benefits of integrating research into clinical care are potentially numerous for the patient, the individual practitioner, and the health care agency.

Before delving into the activities involved in research-based practice, a discussion of how science works and why it is held in high esteem is offered in Chapter 2. Although the content of that chapter can be viewed as supplementary, the issues discussed therein represent the very foundation of research-based practice. In Chapter 3 the overall approach of the book is described in more detail, and various ways of launching research-based practice are discussed. The balance of the book, starting with Chapter 4, covers the pathways of research-based practice and is geared toward providing very specific information relevant to the activities of locating, reading, appraising, and using research evidence.

References

Agency for Health Care Policy and Research, U.S. Department of Health and Human Services. Rockville, MD.

Barlow, D.H., and Hersen, M. (1984). *Single Case Experimental Designs: Strategies for Studying Behavior Change, 2nd edition.* New York: Pergamon.

Cochrane Library (1998). Oxford, UK: Internet address: http://www.cochrane.co.uk

Horsley, J.A., Crane, J., Crabtree, M., and Wood, D. (1983). *Using Research to Improve Nursing Practice: A Guide* [CURN Project]. New York: Grune & Stratton.

Stetler, C.B., and Marram, G. (1976). Evaluating research findings for applicability in practice. *Nursing Outlook, 24,* 559–563.

Science: A Dependable Knowledge Source

Scientists pursue knowledge by establishing investigative conditions under which observations about a particular aspect of reality can be made; then, based on analysis of the observations, they draw conclusions about that reality (i.e., create a conceptual picture of that reality). The conclusions, or the particular picture of reality that is produced, is called a *knowledge claim* (Krathwohl, 1985). Initially, a knowledge claim is evaluated by other specialists in the field based on the scientific soundness of the methods by which it was produced and on whether it is congruent with other established knowledge. Over time, if the findings can be confirmed by replication or by other forms of evidence, the claim is recognized as a true representation of reality.

HUMAN ENTERPRISE

The respect given to science as a way of acquiring knowledge is to a large degree a function of the fact that science acquires, verifies, and builds knowledge through an open, consensus-building process. When a study is completed, a report is generated or a paper is presented at a professional meeting. These presentations enable other people in the field to evaluate the soundness of the methods used, to replicate the study, and ultimately to evaluate the meaning of the findings. To have confidence in the findings, someone else should be able to duplicate the procedure used and obtain the same results. If the knowledge claim is confirmed by other researchers, in different settings, and under slightly different conditions, consensus grows that the knowledge claim provides a plausible portrayal of a particular reality.

Typically, science proceeds via "baby steps," which is to say that studies examine very specific questions and produce knowledge claims that are quite specific. In addition, the open process by which scientific knowledge claims are published and challenged frequently leads to revisions or even retraction of earlier findings; these revisions and retractions should not be viewed as failures of science but recognized as successes, for they are crucial to making forward progress. Thus, science inches forward via a back-and-forth shuffle until a key piece of the knowledge puzzle is discovered. Key discoveries enable scientists to bring prior unfitting pieces of knowledge into association with one another to produce a cohesive explanation of how things work.

An Episode of Science

The case of cold fusion research provides a highly visible portrayal of how science works (Collins and Pinch, 1993). In the late 1980s several groups around the world were trying to establish the conditions under which energy could be created by the fusion of heavy hydrogen atoms. In 1989 two chemists from the University of Utah, Pons and Fleischmann, announced at a press conference that they had succeeded in producing excess heat and nuclear by-product (i.e., neutrons) using apparatus and ingredients available in many modern scientific laboratories. The use of the press conference as a way of announcing this discovery was criticized because the lack of details regarding the methodology and the data made it difficult for other scientists to evaluate the findings. However, the following month a report was published, and the study was presented at an American Physical Society meeting five weeks later. When fusion researchers first heard of Pons and Fleischmann's results they were skeptical because many other scientists had tried to do the same thing and none had succeeded. By the time the meeting of the American Physical Society was held, many scientists working in the field had obtained more details about Pons and Fleischmann's experiment and had tried to replicate the findings. Initially, positive results came in from prestigious university laboratories, but further analysis revealed methodological oversights and measurement errors that could produce inaccurate interpretations. Debate ensued, not the least of which was the argument that the results went against prevailing theory. Over the next several months the credibility of the findings was seriously questioned, and Pons and Fleischmann eventually revised their knowledge claims to a more modest level. This account illustrates the role that open reporting, skepticism, peer review, replication, and theoretical consistency play in evaluating the knowledge claims made by scientists based on one site's results. More important, the account illustrates the self-correcting mechanisms inherent in the scientific process.

Doing the Work of Science

In some sense science is a very conservative social process. Knowledge claims that are unexpected or at odds with current thinking are held to a higher standard of evidence than expected findings; other times findings that are contrary to current thinking may be ignored. For example, in the early 1970s research regarding the role of homocysteine in heart disease was largely ignored because scientists were focused on cholesterol; today a high level of homocysteine (an amino acid) is being recognized as one of the factors that contribute to atherosclerotic plaques.

A radically different way of viewing a particular phenomenon may have difficulty getting serious attention, because scientists in a field have learned to see the phenomena they deal with in a certain way, and that way of seeing can make them blind to other ways of seeing these phenomena. In the 1960s scientists using computers began to pay attention to data that had previously been dismissed as "experimental error" (Gleick, 1987). They came to see a complex order in what had earlier appeared as randomness and unpredictability. With this new vision, they found complex but patterned interacting processes in what other scientists had been taught to ignore. Their theories, collectively referred to as dynamic systems theory, or chaos theory, have produced a radically different way of seeing the processes of everyday physical reality, and are changing the way we think about and study social processes like communication and human behavior.

Another way in which science is self-correcting is that its conclusions are always considered probable, tentative, and open to revision. The most highly regarded thinking in a field today may be revised or even reversed one year from now or 25 years from now if new evidence reveals that the original conclusions were slightly, or even completely, in error. That is, scientists did not accurately capture and convey reality, or they were accurate to a point but failed to uncover more basic processes or the full range of ways in which the phenomenon presents itself. The evolution of scientific knowledge reminds us that even the findings from the latest, largest, and most sophisticated multi-site clinical trial or from a well-conducted meta-analysis must be viewed as tentative, as merely the best evidence we have at this point in time.

Science is certainly not an infallible method for acquiring knowledge. Human ego, ambition, unrecognized bias, theoretical preference, carelessness, and even greed can affect how science is conducted, how questions are framed, how data is obtained, and how the findings are interpreted. Still, it must be acknowledged that scientific research is the most objective and confirmable evidence there is for deciding how to prevent, diagnose, treat, and manage disease, disability, and illness. All other rationales are more prone to being influenced by personal inclination, partial perception, misinterpretation, or faulty reasoning. This is not to say that one's own experiences with patients, advice from colleagues, instruction from a mentor, reasoned action, reliance on recognized authorities, and patients' views should not influence care, but they should always be considered in relation to the scientific evidence available.

POTENTIAL DILEMMAS

A person working within a human service discipline and reading research reports relevant to that discipline will often notice that findings of one study contradict, or at least are substantially different from, those of another study on the same subject. Often the differences can be attributed to differing populations, procedures, or measurement instruments. This attribution is legitimate because research involving human participants is difficult to replicate, that is, to reproduce with precision. However, the consumer of human services research is often faced with the task of trying to make sense of apparently inconsistent findings; guidance for dealing with this issue will be offered in Chapter 9.

Relying on research evidence need not, as some fear, reduce human service practice to the mere application of knowledge. There is still great need and opportunity for personal interpretations and crafting of care. Person-to-person connections need not be diminished just because scientific evidence is given a prominent role in the practitioner's knowledge base. Appreciation of the patient as a unique person, of health care as a collaborative human endeavor, and of expressions of self (e.g., concern, sharing, humor) as essential ingredients of care should still characterize the interpersonal exchange between patient and health care provider.

A huge amount of research is available to health care providers. Historically, scientists in the basic sciences have examined issues such as how lipids are processed in the body; physicians have studied the effectiveness of various ways of treating disease; social scientists have studied issues such as the ways different cultures view aging. Now an increasing amount of research is being done by nurses, rehabilitation and disability specialists, nutritionists, holistic care providers, and other professionals involved in health care. The result of this broad-based input to health care research is that many issues that previously had been ignored are now receiving attention—issues such as the experience of fatigue, quality of life, patient participation in decision making, functional abilities in activities of daily living, and the meaning of chronic illness to family members are being examined from new perspectives. The plethora of research is, of course, a mixed blessing. It's a valuable source of information, but skill and time are required to sort through it, find the most relevant studies, evaluate their meaning, and decide whether or not to change practice. A skill deficit in appraising the research and a lack of time to locate, read, and evaluate studies are two major reasons for what is called the research-practice gap (Pettengill, Gillies, and Clark, 1994).

THE RESEARCH-PRACTICE GAP

Examples

In almost all fields in which research is being conducted, a gap between knowledge production and knowledge utilization exists. The research-practice gap refers to the period that passes from the time when research produces findings that are relevant to practice and the time when they are widely incorporated into practice (Coyle and Sokop, 1990). A recent example of the gap relates to the use of aspirin in preventing acute myocardial infarction and stroke. Depending on what interpretation of the studies you accept, the benefits of aspirin in protecting patients from heart attack and stroke have been known since the mid-1980s. Yet only recently did the U.S. Food and Drug Administration extend their approval of the use of aspirin as a preventive measure in persons who are at high risk for cardiovascular disease but do not have a history of myocardial infarction (MI) or who have stable angina. Previously, aspirin was recommended to reduce the risk of death or a nonfatal myocardial infarction in patients with previous histories of MIs or in those with unstable angina. Thus, the official agency proceeded cautiously even though many primary care providers, based on the studies reported in the medical literature, for years had prescribed aspirin to prevent vascular events in patients without previous MIs whom they viewed to be at risk (Marwick, 1997).

Another interesting example concerns the area of breast cancer research in which a convincing epidemiologic study of the association between regular physical activity and reduced risk of breast cancer has been completed (Thune, Brenn, Lund, and Gaard, 1997). This large prospective study of more than 25,000 Norwegian women resulted in the conclusion that "physical activity during leisure time and at work is associated with a reduced risk of breast cancer" (p. 1269). In an editorial in the same issue (McTiernan 1997), the writer (a physician at a cancer research center) points out that even though this study adds to the evidence from more than a dozen other published studies with similar findings, studies that use better methods of evaluating patterns of activity and that elucidate biological mechanisms need to be conducted before health care providers can tell women that exercise will help prevent breast cancer. Her argument admits that we have considerable strong evidence, but she suggests that important pieces of knowledge are still missing. Some practitioners who read the study or who read this study in combination with others may conclude that the evidence is convincing and that they should take a stronger position on recommending exercise for young women who are at risk for breast cancer. Yet the expert who wrote this editorial expresses a cautionary note for very cogent reasons. She reminds us that to evaluate a correlational finding we must also evaluate the mechanism that brings it about, and at this point in regard to this issue, we cannot do that. The situation demonstrates how difficult it is to decide when the research evidence is sufficient to warrant a change in one's practice.

Reasons for the Gap

The gap between when knowledge is produced and when it is practiced by the majority of potential users occurs for many reasons (Gaus, 1996). Among them, as just discussed, is the wide variance in human nature and in their views of what constitutes "sufficient evidence." When credible research first confirms the advantages of a new way of doing something, it is often not clear exactly who will benefit from the new approach, what the risks are, or how much variation in the approach can be tolerated without affecting the outcomes. A practitioner, or an official agency, may see promise in the findings but is wary of using them because the consequences of using them are not certain, particularly if it would replace a treatment that has been used safely and with seemingly good results. There is always a small group of innovators who will try out new findings as soon as they are made known, but most others hang back and wait for more confirmation (Rogers, 1983). This is not a criticism of the majority, rather a description of the difference in people, as well as a recognition of the wisdom of waiting for several studies with consistent results when one is making recommendations regarding another person's well-being. Ultimately, the practitioner must evaluate research findings in light of the "guesstimated" probability that following the course of action supported by the research will produce desired outcomes for a particular patient or population of patients. What is scientifically possible must be integrated with what is practically doable and acceptable to the patient—this topic will be discussed further in Chapter 7.

Another reason for the delay in using research knowledge is that the people who produce knowledge, i.e., scientists and academic researchers, often associate in different circles and read different professional journals than do practitioners (Mulhall, 1997). As a result, some time may pass between the time a study is completed and when practitioners first become aware of its results—just as time passes between when a clinical question first becomes verbalized and when research into it begins.

The use of different language by researchers and clinicians even when talking about the same issue also impedes the adoption of research findings. For instance, researchers study "bereavement reactions," whereas practitioners talk about patients' depression, overwhelming sadness, and withdrawal. Separate professional circles and different language can reduce the meaningful dialogue between the two groups of people. This is unfortunate, because the lack of dialogue in turn may decrease the relevancy of research efforts as well as slow the use of potentially relevant research findings.

This lack of dialogue is particularly inexpedient because researchers and practitioners share the goals of bringing about better patient outcomes, findings better ways to provide care, and making sense of problematic situations. Argyris and Schon (1996) describe both researchers and practitioners as "inquirers" (p. 36). Researchers systematically and carefully probe situations with the interest of creating dependable explanations for how the world works; practitioners, too, probe situations in the interest of understanding how the world works, albeit with different methods, but they have the additional practical goal of using the knowledge acquired to "design day-to-day strategies of action" (p. 37). Interaction between the two groups of inquirers is essential to achieving their common goal of producing and bringing new knowledge to bear on patient situations.

Too often research is reported in the language of statistics instead of being reported in clinically meaningful terms. Persons who are reporting clinical research need to think in terms of the "end users," i.e., practitioners. For practitioners to have confidence in the research results of a quantitative study, they want to know (a) that the size of the relationship between the variables (e.g., between an intervention and the patient outcome) is clinically meaningful, and (b) that the a statistical relationship of that size does not have a high likelihood of occurring by chance. The first of these issues has to do with the clinical significance of the findings, the second with the statistical significance. The two issues are related but they are not identical; each portrays the results from a different perspective. If only statistical results are reported, the practitioner will be left to decide whether the results of the study are clinically meaningful. There are ways of presenting data as well as some measures of clinical effect that can be included in research reports to assist practitioners in deciding if the findings are clinically meaningful. This issue will be addressed subsequently in Chapters 7, 8, and 10, but for now the point is that one of the factors contributing to a research practice gap is that research reports often do not report data in clinically meaningful forms.

Skill deficits in locating and reading research reports and in appraising research findings are undoubtedly among the reasons for the research-practice gap. Many practitioners currently in practice are many years away from when they took their research and statistics courses. In spite of this, over the years many of these practitioners have continued to build their knowledge of research methodology; however, other practitioners have fallen behind in maintaining research reading and appraisal skills. Even if a practitioner is capable in reading and interpreting research, the time required to locate, read, and critically think about the studies is not always available to many busy health care providers.

The good news regarding the research-practice gap is that clinical journals are publishing research reports with greater frequency, and the reports are written in formats that devote more attention to clinical questions, to the meanings the research findings have for practice, and to the readiness of the findings for practice. The increased presence of useful research reports in clinical journals makes research findings more a part of clinical discourse. In addition, integrative research review articles, in which experts review all the research that has been conducted on a topic and make recommendations for clinical practice, are being published with greater frequency. Practice-focused research conferences also contribute to the discourse by bringing researchers and clinicians together to consider the meaning of findings, their readiness for practice, and the ways in which they could be used in clinical settings (Funk, Tornquist, and Champagne, 1989).

Reverse Gap

The research-practice gap can also work in reverse: practitioners may be aware that information is lacking in a certain area, but it takes quite a while for research to be done and research reports to appear. An example of this was the use of patient-controlled intravenous analgesia. Although some proprietary research had established its safety and general effectiveness and the technology was available and widely used, it took several years for a considerable body of research reports to be published establishing for whom and under what conditions it works best. A more current example is the dearth of research regarding the prevalence and treatment of burns related to the deployment of automobile air safety bags even though emergency care providers are aware of the problem.

Lack of a Gap

Ironically, the lack of a research-practice gap is a problem in some fields, such as AIDS and cancer treatment. In these situations patients and practitioners are eager to use new treatment modalities before scientists studying them consider them ready for use. Even though the benefit of the experimental treatment has not been sufficiently studied to produce confidence in its effectiveness, some people choose to receive experimental treatments because there is no known and tested treatment that would benefit them. These lack-of-gap situations are extraordinary and create a whole set of dilemmas that are not examined in this book.

SUMMARY

In summary, scientific research is a process by which knowledge is extracted from the real world. This process serves as a valuable tool in the search for knowledge, but it does not set us on a direct path to knowledge; rather, it is a path that inherently involves stumbling, that is, making mistakes followed by correcting those mistakes. Sometimes the correction occurs within months; other times it takes many years. Science moves toward knowledge via a slow, laborious zigzag. Single studies are small steps on that zigzag, and must be viewed with skepticism. The research utilization process organizes skepticism into a systematic and critical appraisal of single studies and subsequently of a group of studies. Those appraisals help the practitioner determine whether to incorporate changes in the way he or she does something.

References

Argyris, C., and Schon, D.A. (1996). *Organizational Learning II: Theory, Method and Practice.* Reading, MA: Addison-Wesley.

Collins, H., and Pinch, T. (1993). *The Golem: What Everyone Should Know about Science.* Cambridge: University Press.

Coyle, L.A., and Sokop, A.G. (1990). Innovation adoption behavior among nurses. *Nursing Research, 39*:176–181.

Funk, S.G., Tornquist, E.M., and Champagne, M.T. (1989). Application and evaluation of the dissemination model. *Western Journal of Nursing Research, 11*:486–491.

Gaus, C.R. (1996). *Quality Health Care and the Role of Health Services Research: Testimony by the Administrator of the Agency for Health Care Policy and Research before a hearing of the Senate Appropriations Subcommittee on Labor, HHS and Education,* November 13, 1996.

Gleick, J. (1987). *Chaos: Making a New Science.* New York: Penguin.

Krathwohl, D.R. (1985). *Social and Behavioral Science Research.* San Francisco: Jossey-Bass.

Marwick, C. (1997). Aspirin's role in prevention now official. *Journal of the American Medical Association, 277*:701–702.

McTiernan, A. (1997). *Editorial: Exercise and breast cancer—A time to get moving? The New England Journal of Medicine, 336*:1311–1312.

Mulhall, A. (1997). Nursing research: Our world not theirs. *Journal of Advanced Nursing, 25*:969–976.

Rogers, E.M. (1983). *Diffusion of Innovations,* 3rd ed. New York: Free Press.

Thune, I., Brenn, T., Lund, E., and Gaard, M. (1997). Physical activity and the risk of breast cancer. *The New England Journal of Medicine,* 336:1269–1275.

Getting Started

Research-based practice starts with a practitioner, or a group of care providers, recognizing a need for research-based knowledge in a particular situation. The process then advances to an appraisal of the available research evidence and a decision regarding whether and how to change practice, and ends with an evaluation of whether the research-based change in practice actually did benefit patients. Although this description makes research-based practice seem like a direct, even linear, process, the reality is that there are several pathways connecting the starting points to the end point. The pathways, which are illustrated in Figure 3–1, provide the practitioner with several options regarding how to proceed with research-based practice. This map of the research-based practice pathways will be used throughout the book to orient the reader to the pathway or steps being addressed in a particular chapter. One or several boxes will be shaded to indicate the topic of the chapter—this shading will serve the same function as a "You are here" X on trail and mall maps.

The pathways contained in the research-based practice strategy of this book extend and combine ideas from many sources that have addressed the critique and use of research findings. Foremost among them is the influence of the nursing profession's long-standing interest in the use of research in practice (Haller, Reynolds, and Horsley, 1979) and the more recent approaches developed by the evidence-based medicine movement (Sackett, Richardson, Rosenberg, and Haynes, 1997). The emphasis on the clinical significance of findings gained substance from the writings of Rosnow and Rosenthal (1993) on the difference between statistical and practical significance. The pathway for the appraisal of collective evidence reflects the work on integrative reviews by Cooper (1982), by Cooper and Hedges (1994), and by the Agency for Health Care Policy and Research of the U.S. Department of Health and Human Services. The emphasis on the applicability of findings to a particular setting owes a great deal to the Stetler/Marram model for the application of research findings to practice (Stetler, 1994). Other components of the Stetler/Marram model that influenced the approach of this book include (a) taking into account the basis and effectiveness of current practice, (b) the need to have more solid evidence when risk to the patient is possible, and (c) recognition of different ways in which research can influence practice.

Pathways of Research-based Practice

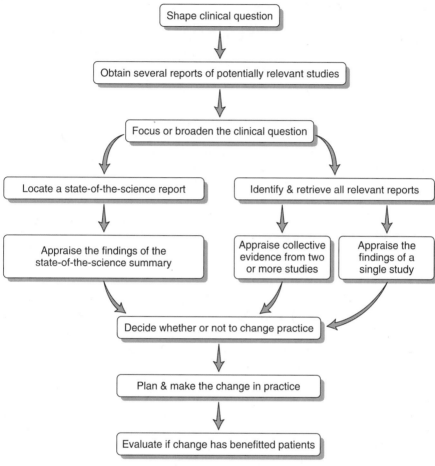

Figure 3–1.

PATHWAYS OF RESEARCH-BASED PRACTICE

Three Distinct Pathways

Research-based practice can progress along three distinct pathways. All three pathways start with the identification of a clinical question of interest, and proceed to a search for potentially relevant research evidence (i.e., original studies, summaries of prior research, or research-based guidelines). Depending on how much research has been done about the topic, the original question may be revised to narrow or broaden its focus at this point. Having completed these two steps, you will also know what kind of evidence is available, and that will influence the pathway of research-based practice you will take from there. The pathway choices are (1) appraisal of the findings of a state-of-the-science summary, (2) appraisal of the collective evidence from two or more studies, and (3) appraisal of the findings from a single research study. (State-of-the-science summaries can take the form of a meta-analysis, an integrative research review, or a research-based guideline.)

Regardless of which pathway you choose, if you make a change in practice based on the research evidence, you should plan some way of evaluating whether the research-based practice you implemented has benefited your patients. Therefore, it is recommended that after the change has been in place for a period of time, you evaluate its effect on your patients using some form of quality improvement data. Evaluating the effects of your changes is discussed further in Chapter 11.

Choosing a Pathway

There is no one right pathway; rather, the "best" pathway will be the one that is appropriate to the type and amount of research evidence available and is feasible given your time and resources. The pathway involving the use of findings from a state-of-the-science summary is the way of proceeding with the potential to bring the greatest amount of research evidence to bear on a question with the least amount of time and effort on your part. In essence, the author of the summary report will have brought together the findings from many, often all, studies on an issue or question. However, it's not a matter of simply extracting the findings from the summary report and transferring them to your practice. You should critically appraise them for credibility and applicability to your setting. This appraisal will require a modicum of skills in reading research summaries, as they do employ unique assumptions, techniques, language, and statistics, all of which will be addressed in Chapter 10.

If in reviewing the literature you cannot locate a state-of-the-science summary report, or if the one you find is not credible, you should locate the reports of all potentially relevant individual studies,[1] and appraise the evidence from them collectively, a process that is sometimes called an across-studies appraisal. Your judgment regarding the strength of the collective evidence will determine if and how you decide to change your practice. The collective-evidence pathway often requires more time than the other two pathways, but it allows a change of practice to be based on a broader scope of information than using a single study. Depending on your topic and on

---

[1] A modulation of the "all" part of this statement will be offered in Chapter 9, but "*all* potentially relevant studies" should be the ideal standard for appraising the evidence regarding a clinical question.

the number of studies that have been conducted relevant to it, you may have just a few or a large number of studies to review and appraise—when the latter is the case, considerable time will be involved.

When only one study has been done on the topic or you only have time to appraise the findings of one study, these realities will dictate that you take the single-study pathway. The skills required to appraise the findings of a single study are the easiest to learn, and appraisal of a single study usually requires less time than the other two pathways; however, it also has the disadvantage of providing a limited basis for making a change in practice.

In this text, the sequence of presentation of the pathways starts with the findings of a single study (Chapter 8), proceeds to collective evidence (Chapter 9), and ends with the findings of a state-of-the-science summary (Chapter 10), even though the recommended order for practitioners engaging in research-based practice is the reverse. The rationale for the presentation sequence is that the issues involved in appraisal of the findings of a single study serve as a foundation for the more complex issues involved in appraising collective evidence and the findings of a state-of-the-science summary. Hence, the sequence of presentation accommodates the learning process rather than the recommended order of use of the three pathways.

GETTING REAL

Although the research-based practice strategy described in this book upholds the standard of performing a systematic appraisal of *all* research reports relevant to a clinical question, accommodations to the realities of time expenditure may have to be accepted. It is important to note that the use of a good, recent state-of-the-science summary does not represent a compromise from that standard, as such summaries often review all the research on a topic. There may be times, however, when your database search does not locate a state-of-the-science summary but does identify two or more studies on your topic—and you just don't have the time to read all of them. You may have to take the appraisal-of-a-single-study pathway even though you know the appraisal-of-collective-evidence pathway would yield more complete evidence. You would, of course, try to read the study that most directly addresses your clinical question and does so using a sample similar to the patient(s) you have in mind. Unbiased ways for reducing the number of studies you read and appraise are presented in Chapter 9, in which appraisal of collective evidence is discussed, but for now the point is that you may have to learn to accept using the a single-study pathway even though you know the better way would be to use the collective-evidence pathway. Clearly, basing your practice on the findings from one study has advantages over not basing it on any research at all.

Hypothetical Situation

Consider the following situation: You are on the health advisory board of a senior citizen center that will be offering an influenza and pneumonia vaccination clinic in the fall; the board will be discussing how to increase participation over last year's level. In preparing for this meeting, if you spend 15 minutes doing a search at the PubMed (Medline) query site, which is available on the Internet through the National Institutes of Health, using the search terms "influenza vaccination," "elderly," and "acceptance," you would find citations and some abstracts for 20 to 30 relevant studies. You obviously can't thoroughly appraise all of them just to prepare for the meeting, but let's say in browsing the abstracts you are struck by how frequently primary care providers' recommendations to elderly patients to have a vaccination have been found to determine whether they actually get flu shots or not (Fiebach and Viscoli, 1991; Ganguly and Webster, 1995; Nichol, MacDonald and Hauge, 1996). Based on this preliminary information, you tentatively decide that you would like to recommend to the board that a letter be written to local providers telling them about the clinic and reminding them to tell their high-risk clients about it. Because you have limited time, you decide to pick out two reports that address this aspect of the issue, and obtain the original reports of those studies from your local health science library. If your appraisal of them determines that they were soundly conducted and the findings are applicable to your situation, you will have strong, objective information on which to base your recommendation that a letter be sent to local providers. Not only can the research-based information be used at the board meeting, but you might also want to cite the studies in the letter to providers reminding them of how important their recommendations are.

Had you not browsed the research literature, you might not have realized how influential provider recommendations are in determining whether or not elderly persons get vaccinated. Thus, even though you did not conduct a systematic and exhaustive review of all the research regarding the role of provider recommendations in influencing whether or not a person gets a flu shot, your practice will be more research-based than if you had not searched the available research at all. The standard of using all available research evidence when determining a course of action needs to remain in place, particularly for a course of action that involves risk to the patient, but most assuredly it can be modulated at times.

The problem with not using all studies is that you may be omitting findings from other studies that contradict the studies you are using or that identify conditions under which the findings do not hold up. In other words, your sample of two studies may not be representative of the entire evidence base relevant to the issue; it may be biased. You should be less confident about using the findings from two studies than you would be about using findings from the entire evidence base of studies related to designing an influenza and pneumonia vaccination program. Still, using two studies would provide the board with a better basis for designing a marketing strategy than would not considering any research at all.

Assessing Your Knowledge Base

Another aspect of "getting real" involves objectively assessing your ability, or the collective ability of your group, to appraise research reports, a collection of studies on a topic, and systematic summaries of research. Although clinical knowledge is an important requirement for appraising research and considering how to translate findings into practice, knowledge of research terminology, design, and statistics is also necessary. As an individual, you may feel a need to attend a continuing education workshop on evidence-based practice offered by one of your professional organizations, or enroll in a research or statistics course at a local community college. If you feel you have a deficit in the skills required for searching the databases of health care literature, you could remedy this by scheduling time with the librarian at the hospital or by attending a workshop on how to use a particular search engine or database. Any time invested in developing your research or statistics knowledge or your database searching skills will enhance your ability to locate, read, and appraise research evidence, and will most likely also save you time and frustration as you proceed with research-based practice. Perhaps the only preparation you require is to purchase a current health science research text, or possibly a statistics text, to use as a reference source when reading research reports. Several good texts are cited in the references at the end of Chapter 7.

To ensure that studies are correctly and fully understood, most groups made up primarily of clinicians will benefit from having a health care researcher available during discussions. The researcher will be able to explain the more complex aspects of design and analysis and to add specialized research knowledge to the discussions. If a researcher is not available, a person who has had several research courses and has an interest and experience in the appraisal and use of research findings should be invited to join the group. The effort expended to identify and invite such a person will undoubtedly be well worth the effort in terms of perspective added to the group's discussion and the added depth of information relevant to appraising the credibility of the findings.

GROUP APPROACHES

Advantages to a Group Approach

Some practitioners may be able to enter into a research-based practice project with colleagues, whereas others will have to rely on their own individual initiative. There are advantages to approaching research-based practice as a member of a group, particularly a multidisciplinary group. The group could be loosely goal-oriented, like a journal club that is reading research articles to increase their comfort with research reports and at the same time get new ideas for patient care in a particular clinical speciality. Alternatively, the group may be highly purposeful such as a task force charged with deciding whether a new approach to care should be adopted, a multidisciplinary group charged with developing a clinical pathway, or a hospital standards committee committed to basing clinical care policies on available research. Somewhere in between is the group practice or multidisciplinary group of providers in a clinical care program who are attempting to move toward research-based practice by implementing a research-based guideline that has been developed by a national health care organization.

Depending on the nature of the group, the level of skill in appraising research studies of its members, and its purpose, several reports could be assigned for everyone to read and appraise, or members could be assigned different reports to read and report on. Having several people read the same study can be very helpful, particularly at the beginning of a research-based practice initiative, because each person will see different aspects, strengths, and weakness in the study, as well as different meaning and implications in the results. Thus, discussion of the report can serve to help develop everyone's research reading and appraisal skills.

Beginning efforts at reading and appraising research reports may be most easily and safely done in a group made up of people from the same discipline—the commonality of perspective and language, as well as the absence of multidisciplinary deference and domination behaviors, can enhance learning and increase risk taking by group members. Once members of a group have acquired skills in appraising research reports, they will be more comfortable being the only person to appraise a report and report the findings to the group as well as more comfortable being a contributing member of a multidisciplinary group.

A Multidisciplinary Approach

In a multidisciplinary group each person could assume responsibility for examining a different aspect of the problem. For example, in considering how to structure a counseling program for families who have a member with Alzheimer's disease, each person in the group would be responsible for identifying and retrieving the research pertaining to the clinical problems she manages. A nurse could look into research describing how families perceive the burden of care for spouses and parents and the factors that determine families' perception of burden of care. The physical therapist could review exercise programs, and the nutritionist could examine the research related to eating problems and their management. A physician could look at pharmacological management of several common problems, and the occupational therapist could review and appraise studies examining how home environments can be adapted to maximize the functioning and safety of the person with the disease. By using such an approach, this group could develop a counseling program that is comprehensive and broadly research-based.

GETTING LAUNCHED

Research-based practice involves establishing professional values as much as a way of practicing. You have to be convinced that it is a better way of practicing, and you have to commit to it. As with your personal values, your commitment has to be lived out over time and put into action through planning and effort. Time dedicated to research-based practice must be blocked off in advance and honored when the time comes; then you just need to dig in and start doing it. Effort will be required to persist through the frustrations that inevitably accompany learning new skills. However, as suggested in Chapter 2, the payoffs that result for you and your patients will undoubtedly compensate for the effort.

Starting Points

Research-based practice can be launched from one of two starting points (Titler et al., 1994). One starting point is scanning journals for research that could be applicable to practice and then, after consideration of its merit, incorporating the findings into practice. In contrast, another starting point originates in practice itself, with the practitioner recognizing the need for more or better information about an issue, and proceeds to a purposeful search of the literature for relevant research. Even though the problem-solving starting point seems more purposeful, sometimes one doesn't realize that there is an alternative way of doing something; thus, the scanning approach has the potential to increase one's awareness of the need or the existence of new knowledge. The emphasis in this book is on the problem-solving starting point because it often leads to consideration of more than one study; however, both starting points play an important role in improving practice.

Spurs to Research-Based Practice

Most of us change our behavior because there is some spur that enters our lives, either once in a dramatic way or repeatedly in a persistent manner, reminding us that we need to change the way we do things. In professional health care practice that spur may be a situation in which you felt you didn't have the knowledge to address a patient's question well, even though you should have. Or a clinical situation may keep recurring, and you believe that your way of dealing with it is less than optimal.

A nurse practitioner reported that she felt she never had a helpful and specific answer when healthy, middle-aged patients asked her about what kind of exercise they should be doing. She felt she needed to find out what research evidence there was about the benefits of aerobic exercise, stretching, and weight training for healthy people and how often they should engage in them to experience benefits. The initial results of her literature search and how she focused her questions will be presented in the next chapter, but the point here is that she was sensitive to her inadequate knowledge base and didn't just try to get by with general, lay press knowledge. She made a real effort to get research evidence on which to base her counsel to her patients.

Sometimes the spur to finding out what the research has to say about a clinical issue is the initiation of a new clinical protocol, program, or clinical pathway. We have this sense that new beginnings deserve a fresh outlook and the best basis possible, so new clinical initiatives provide an incentive to be as research-based as possible in what we recommend. Another spur is when a quality improvement monitoring report provides feedback indicating that patients are not satisfied with a particular aspect of care or that patients are not achieving the outcomes that clinical pathways set forth for them. Regardless of what spurs you to consider whether looking at the research would provide valuable evidence to guide future action, the next step is to think clearly and specifically about what you need to know.

SUMMARY

Getting started in research-based practice requires commitment, time, and research knowledge. Unfortunately, none of these commodities are easy to come by in most health care settings. Professional providers are reluctant to make new commitments, even to activities they believe are valuable, because their days are already so busy. Most providers value research-based knowledge and would like to incorporate it into their practice, but many of them are overwhelmed by the volume of studies published or by the demands required to read and evaluate the relevant evidence.

Realistically, research-based practice cannot be achieved "on the run"—it requires time to ascertain what evidence has been produced, time to carefully read and appraise the evidence, and time to think about and decide whether to make a change in practice. To read a research report or a summary of research studies and truly understand the question asked, how the study was done, and what the findings were often requires an hour or more. In addition, many providers are not confident that they can read a research report and know whether it was well enough conducted to trust its results. Thus, time may also be required to develop the necessary appraisal knowledge and skills.

To avoid paralysis, first you need to realize that the necessary knowledge and skills can be acquired incrementally over time—they don't have to be entirely in your possession at the beginning of the endeavor. Second, an hour per week spent on locating, reading, and appraising research evidence will have a significant impact on your practice. Third, if possible, you should embark on research-based practice in the company of others. Attempting to go it alone may result in discouragement, whereas engaging in it with others will undoubtedly make the learning and the appraisal of the evidence more productive as well as more enjoyable.

Most groups of practitioners embarking on research-based practice will benefit greatly from inviting or contracting with a health care researcher to work with them in appraising the research evidence. In most situations, the technical knowledge the researcher brings to the discussion will enrich the appraisal of the evidence considerably. Finally, even though these investments of time and effort may seem demanding, you may need to remind yourself that failure to make the investment will result in care that is out-of-date or less than the best possible. Investing in research-based practice will bring important benefits to your patients and to you in the form of professional satisfaction in the long run.

References

Agency for Health Care Policy and Research, U.S. Department of Health and Human Services. Rockville, MD.

Cooper, H.M. (1982). Scientific guidelines for conducting integrative research reviews. *Review of Educational Research, 52*:291–302.

Cooper, H., and Hedges, L.V. (eds.) (1994). *The Handbook of Research Synthesis.* New York: Russell Sage Foundation.

Fiebach, N.H., and Viscoli, C.M. (1991). Patient acceptance of influenza vaccination. *American Journal of Medicine, 91*:393–400.

Ganguly, R., and Webster, T.B. (1995). Influenza vaccination in the elderly. *Journal of Investigational Allergology and Clinical Immunology, 5*:73–77.

Haller, K.B., Reynolds, M.A., and Horsley, J.A. (1979). Developing research-based innovation protocols: Process, criteria, and issues. *Research in Nursing and Health, 2*:45–51.

Nichol, K.L., MacDonald, R., and Hauge, M. (1996). Factors associated with influenza and pneumococcal vaccination behavior among high-risk adults. *Journal of General Internal Medicine, 11*:673–677.

Rosnow, R.L., and Rosenthal, R. (1993). *Beginning Behavioral Research: A Conceptual Primer.* New York: Macmillan.

Sackett, D.L., Richardson, W.S., Rosenberg, W., and Haynes, R.B. (1997). *Evidence-Based Medicine: How to Practice & Teach EBM.* New York: Churchill Livingstone.

Stetler, C.B. (1994). Refinement of the Stetler/Marram model for application of research findings to practice. *Nursing Outlook, 42*:15–25.

Titler, M.G., Kleiber, C., Steelman, V., Goode, C., Rakel, B., Barry-Walker, J., Small, S., and Buckwalter, K. (1994). Infusing research into practice to promote quality care. *Nursing Research, 43*:307–313.

4

Shaping the Clinical Question

Most clinical questions have their origins in the patient-provider encounter or in the clinical thinking of the provider as he deliberates about what care to offer a patient or population of patients. Other questions are formulated during professional dialogue or while examining and discussing quality improvement data. In this chapter the original formulation of a clinical question and its re-formulation after the practitioner has browsed the research base on the topic are considered (see Figure 4–1).

Clinical questions originate in the minds of reflective practitioners. The practitioner who is on automatic pilot when providing care will not see patterns in her practice indicating that some approach is not working well, will not acknowledge that she lacks knowledge regarding how to treat a particular patient, and will not seek out research to use in daily practice. In contrast, the reflective practitioner will come away from everyday practice with several questions asking how, what, when, who, or why:

- What nonpharmacological measures are effective for managing affected-side muscle spasms in post-stroke patients?
- Why do some adolescent girls in poor, urban neighborhoods not get pregnant?
- Should I recommend nutritional supplements to my elderly patients for improved immunity?
- If a patient asks about the risk of missed dental disease when she elects to not have mouth x-rays done at the time of a full-mouth examination, what can I tell her?
- Are once-a-day vital signs adequate in hospitalized, nonsurgical adult patients when compared to four-times-a-day vital signs?
- What social situations are most troublesome to suburban families with one or more members who are HIV positive?
- What factors determine whether middle-aged men working in an industrial plant continue back reinjury prevention exercises instituted at the time of an injury?

FOCUS

Noticeably, the foregoing questions are focused; they are not vague. In each of these questions, a specific "who" is named, and one or more phenomena of interest are specified. Most often an area of interest is a health outcome (i.e., freedom from affected-side muscle spasm, missed dental disease, improved immunity, not pregnant). Frequently, one of the phenomena is an

Pathways of Research-based Practice

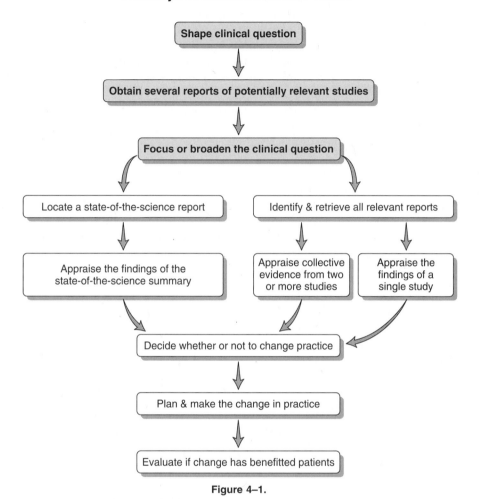

Figure 4–1.

intervention (i.e., nonpharmacological management, not having dental x-rays, back reinjury prevention exercise program). In some questions, a comparison between two interventions may constitute the element in question (e.g., the vital sign question), and in others a time frame or setting (e.g., in an industrial plant) may be of interest. In fact, each of these questions could probably be stated even more specifically by a practitioner who deals with the problem every day because she would know exactly which aspects of the questions are particularly troublesome or questionable.

Your clinical questions must be focused because most research by its very nature is directed at specific questions. Overall, research is aimed at understanding whether a specific phenomenon exists, how it works, what effects it has, and under what conditions it works. In order to fully answer all the questions about something, however, a series of studies must be conducted. Any single research study can only examine one or two aspects of the overall issue. The question "Are once-a-day vital signs adequate in hospitalized, nonsurgical adult patients when compared with four-times-a-day vital signs?" is an example of a question that is focused from a hospital staff's point of view, but is not framed in a way in which such research is likely to be found. From a research perspective, it is too broad, and it contains several questions. To collect research evidence about "vital signs" there are four groups of studies that need to be considered: studies regarding temperature fluctuations and elevations, another regarding heart rate patterns and changes, another about blood pressure determinations, and a fourth about respiratory patterns and rates. A research study is more likely to address the requisite frequency of one of the four parameters rather than all four, because addressing all of them would introduce the need for many control subjects, many populations, and many outcome variables—all of which would make a very complex study. Even though care providers eventually need answers to the more general question pertaining to once-a-day vital signs, they must realize that from a research perspective, the question contains four research questions. The job of pulling the separate research bases together to answer the real world question must be done by the end user of research, i.e., the practitioner.

Another example of a clinical question that must be broken down into more specific questions when appraising its research base is a question regarding outcomes associated with cardiac rehabilitation. Cardiac rehabilitation is not a discrete intervention; rather, it is an amalgam of interventions composed of graduated aerobic exercising, education about stress reduction, education about managing the disease, counseling about living with heart disease, dietary education, weight loss, and smoking cessation. Although it is possible to study the effects of a total program, the research would be of limited value because other sites would not be able to duplicate the entire program with precision. More important, nothing would be learned about which components are associated with what outcomes. Thus, research is more likely to proceed by examining the effects of each of the components of cardiac rehabilitation separately, before considering how they work in combination. When formulating a clinical question, you must give some thought to how research on the issue might have been done. Fortunately, if you fail to do this in your initial formulation of the question, when you start searching the databases for studies, you will soon realize that you are really asking several questions, not just one. In that way, you will begin to adjust your focus.

Adjusting the Focus

Having said that a clinical question for research evidence should be focused, it also needs to be acknowledged that there is a place for broader questions, particularly when one is first learning about an issue. Consider the question: What are the effects on children of having a parent with a chronic debilitating illness? Even though the question doesn't name the kinds of effects, the age of the children, or a chronic illness of interest, the question does represent a beginning effort to acquire knowledge about an issue one knows little about. If your literature search produces a large number of studies, you may decide to narrow the question to young children or to social adjustment and school problems. or you may decide to focus on chronic diseases involving severe activity restrictions. Often 15 minutes browsing the databases on a topic will give you a good sense of what research has been done, and will enable you to change your clinical question to a form that is answerable by available research evidence. An alternative approach to narrowing your question would be to go to a textbook and read about the problems, and then use that knowledge to formulate a more specific question.

If you ask your question too specifically at the beginning and find no studies that address it, you will have to broaden your question, or you may have to settle for research that is related to the question but does not directly address it. For example, the question above about continuing back reinjury prevention exercises may be too specific, and you may not be able to locate reports directly pertaining to it. As result, you may have to settle for a mix of studies about the factors that influence whether middle-aged men in general exercise on an ongoing basis, why persons with back problems commit to ongoing back exercises, and the overall effectiveness of back health programs in industrial health settings. The answer to your original question may have to be an amalgam of findings put together from several different studies, each bearing to a limited extent, or indirectly, on your question.

A Short Case History of Focusing

In Chapter 3 a nurse practitioner who was seeking information related to advising healthy middle-aged adults about how to exercise was introduced. To develop an answerable question, this nurse practitioner accessed PubMed via the Internet and entered the terms "exercise and middle age" and came up with approximately 28,000 documents! She then narrowed the search using techniques that will be discussed in Chapter 5. Still, she found no research that addressed a program of aerobic exercise, stretch exercise, and strength training (there were many studies examining the effects of one of the three forms). The search also produced many studies that were specific to the role of exercise in managing a particular health problem, such as diabetes or hypertension, but she eliminated these because she was interested in healthy adults who wanted to exercise for general fitness and health purposes. Also, even though she had specified "middle age" in her search, many studies examined the effects of exercise in elderly persons. Some studies addressed "aging"; she decided these studies could be related to her interest, as middle-aged people are interested in promoting healthy aging. Finally, quite a few studies compared alterations in body composition and exercise capacity associated with aging in sedentary and regularly exercising adults; somewhat arbitrarily, she decided she was more interested in interventions than in the aging process itself.

At this point the nurse practitioner realized she needed to refocus her question. In the process of searching she had found several review articles about the effects of aerobic exercising and it seemed clear that there is considerable research documenting its benefits, as well as wide consensus regarding its benefits and its specifics (U.S. Department of Health and Human Services, 1996). Stretching and weight training, also called resistance training, seemed less clear. Stretching, she felt, has a large common-sense piece to it, so again arbitrarily, she decided to focus her quest on the effects of weight training on middle-aged persons and found ten recent studies, which she decided to appraise.

She pointed out that there were many more studies on the effects of weight training in the elderly, and that many of these have indirect relevance to middle-aged persons. This whole process of narrowing her questions took about 45 minutes, using PubMed, but in addition to narrowing her question she also became aware of other issues related to exercise and aging that affected her clinical thinking. She became aware of the importance of noticing body composition when examining middle-aged and older adults, talking with middle-aged adults about the decreased energy usage associated with aging, and discussing the value of walking with older adults. She later stated that she found the process of accessing a large number of abstracts on the subject of exercise and aging to be informative in and of itself. Even though she would not be systematically evaluating the research base on them, she reminded herself that she should be talking with patients about them because they are no- to low-risk forms of advice with considerable research support. This case illustrates how the step of formulating a clinical question is not separate from the step of searching the databases for potentially relevant studies—your original clinical question will undoubtedly undergo change as you get into a database.

Elements of the Clinical Question

The clinical questions for which practitioners seek research evidence are quite diverse, so it is difficult to state exactly what elements (variables, if you prefer) should make up the question. However, a well-formed question typically includes at least three of the elements displayed in Box 4–1. Inclusion of too many elements produces a question that may be so narrow that relevant studies will not be found, whereas consideration of just one element produces a general topic, not a question. Most often, if a topic is too broad, the search will generate a large number of studies that have little in common.

COMPOSITION OF THE RESEARCH EVIDENCE

Some questions are specific, and research directly pertaining to them will be available. For example, a search related to the question of how much blood should be discarded when drawing samples for coagulation studies

---

Box 4–1

Elements of a Clinical Question

- A clinical outcome
- An intervention or treatment; a comparison intervention or treatment
- A preventive or diagnostic action
- A patient experience
- A population of interest; a comparison population
- Associated factors (e.g., beliefs, traits, states, social influences)
- A time factor or a setting

---

from a heparinized arterial catheter will produce studies that directly and specifically answer this question. Other questions may seem as specific, but when you start looking at the studies, you will realize that each study addresses just one or two aspects of the question rather than addressing the question comprehensively. For example, "How should orthostatic hypotension be evaluated?" is a specific question, but each study will not address all important aspects of the question. Some research pertains to the timing of the measurement in relation to meals so as to be able to differentiate between positional (orthostatic) hypotension and hypoglycemic hypotension; some studies examine timing of the measurement from the perspective of how long the person should be standing before taking the measurement; and other research addresses the timing related to when the person last took cardiac and blood pressure medications. To answer the original question, one would have to look at the findings from all three types of studies and put together an answer that is a composite of all three aspects of evaluating orthostatic hypotension.

Finally, it may be necessary to accept the fact that sometimes research has not been done that directly and specifically answers your question; as a result, you may have to assemble an answer on the basis of research from similar but not identical populations, from animal studies, or from studies of related issues. One nurse who was interested in the effects of nicotine withdrawal on patients who stay in the hospital for three or four days after having surgery was not able to locate studies that directly addressed this question. Instead, she obtained and appraised studies examining the effects of nicotine withdrawal on cognitive states, experiences, and performance. Then she made inferences as to how these findings might affect postoperative patients in particular. Granted, she had to make a bit of a leap, but still she was basing her practice on what is known about the effects of nicotine withdrawal on cognition and physical well-being.

QUESTIONS RESEARCH CANNOT ANSWER

To be answerable by research findings, a clinical question asks about what is, about what something is like, about how something works, or about the effects of something. Research can also provide relevant information to use in deciding what should be done, but cannot directly answer questions that involve choosing between values or choosing a moral or ethical course of action. These are questions for philosophical inquiry, not for science. Thus, research cannot answer questions such as the following: Should I aggressively treat the pneumonia of patients in nursing homes who are over 90 years old, and are deaf, blind, or bed-ridden? Is it ethical to not treat the respiratory difficulty of a newborn infant with multiple defects due to trisomy 18? Research can produce information about survival rates and the quality of life associated with various levels of treatment for these two situations, but cannot directly answer the question of what one should do in a particular situation.

SUMMARY

Designing a clinical question that will serve as the basis for an examination of the research literature involves striking a balance between specificity and broadness. If the question is designed too narrowly, you will not be able to find studies directly addressing it. However, if you design it too broadly, you will be faced with a large number of studies to evaluate. As a result, you may need to use the "grope method," particularly when you are new in asking these kinds of questions. First, design the question as it makes sense to you clinically. Specify at least one variable of interest, possibly two, and a population of interest. If a time frame, setting, or comparison seems important, include it. Then search for studies that directly pertain to your question. If you find too few or too many studies, either broaden your question or narrow it (e.g., drop or add the population requirement from your search) to produce a question for which there is a reasonable number of studies to evaluate. Finally, be prepared to accept the possibility that the research available may not answer your clinical question as directly as you would like, but still can be used to design practice that is based on research envidence.

References

U.S. Department of Health and Human Services (1996). *Physical Activity and Health: A Report of the Surgeon General.* Pittsburgh: Superintendent of Documents.

5

Searching for Studies

Fred Pond

LAUNCHING YOUR SEARCH

Getting Started

When beginning your search for studies, it is a good idea to begin searching in a broad and open manner rather than starting very specifically (see Figure 5–1). Searching broadly will be particularly helpful if you are in doubt about how to state your clinical question. Begin by briefly identifying the indexes, journals, and other knowledge sources of which you are aware, and spend some time perusing them. Don't worry about being comprehensive at this point. Rather, take the approach that you are surveying the literature to develop a sense for the specialized language and the breadth of studies that have been done on your topic.

Try to obtain a sense of the maturity of the literature on the topic. Do the article titles address introductory or new-approach themes, or do they review long-established, well-known information? Are the studies that have been done exploratory or is the research at the stage where field trials are being conducted? If you are delving into an area that is completely new to you, books might be an alternative place to begin. Books usually contain accepted, standard knowledge, whereas journals report newer approaches and developments.

While getting familiar with the field and with your topic, keep track of the various terms under which your topic may be identified and the different aspects of the topic on which studies have been done. Strive to become aware of synonyms as well as broader and narrower terms that relate to your topic. When you start to do your search you may find that the literature indexes refer to your topic in a formal manner, instead of the terms that are used in everyday clinical discussions. For example, CPR will be identified

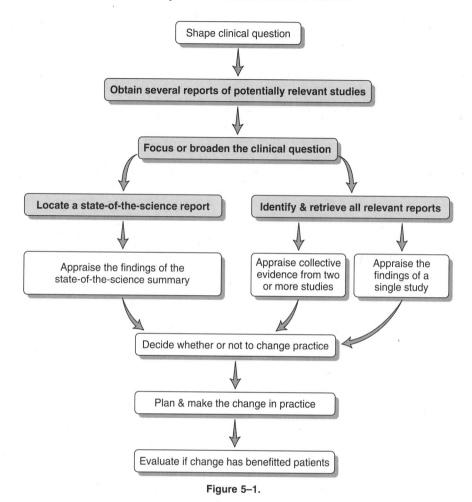

Pathways of Research-based Practice

Shape clinical question

Obtain several reports of potentially relevant studies

Focus or broaden the clinical question

Locate a state-of-the-science report

Identify & retrieve all relevant reports

Appraise the findings of the state-of-the-science summary

Appraise collective evidence from two or more studies

Appraise the findings of a single study

Decide whether or not to change practice

Plan & make the change in practice

Evaluate if change has benefitted patients

Figure 5–1.

as cardiopulmonary resuscitation, not by its abbreviation. In summary, during your brief survey of available resources you should begin to develop an understanding of how your topic appears in the literature, what disciplines are most likely to be writing about it, and where it is likely to be indexed (Dumas, Shurpin, and Gallo, 1995).

Working with a Librarian

Shortly after beginning your project you should consider contacting a health sciences librarian or the reference librarian who is responsible for the literature of your clinical discipline. Ask for an appointment to discuss your research-based practice objectives, rather than talking at the busy reference desk of the library where the emphasis is on providing quick directions and brief instruction. Share your overall concept and approach to your topic. It is not necessary to have a complete idea of your approach at this point. The librarian can give you pointers to help you get started, and will be able to act as a consultant as you proceed.

You could, of course, tell the librarian what your question is and ask him to perform the search or pay a commercial search service to perform it. This approach may seem like the easiest way to identify relevant studies, but a great deal will be lost if you do not participate in the search yourself. You understand the topic and the specific aspects of it in which you are interested and you have clinical knowledge to bring to bear on the search; the librarian typically does not. In addition, during the search practitioners often reshape their questions or change them somewhat; if a librarian does the search, the question is not apt to evolve. A logical compromise, therefore, is for you and the librarian to sit down together in order to combine his searching knowledge and skills with your clinical knowledge.

COMPUTERIZED SEARCHING

Your topic will dictate the actual methods or process you use to find studies. Generally, however, there are two options: (1) manual searching of printed indexes, catalogs, books, and journals; and (2) computerized online searches of electronic indexes or databases. The emphasis in this chapter is on computerized searches, as most health care providers have access to one or more computerized database systems. For those who do not, a discussion of manual searching is provided in Appendix A.

The advent of computer literature searching has made locating research studies, summaries, and research-based practice guidelines a great deal easier. The user can search library catalogs electronically to access health science references from as far back as the 1960s, and can even read electronic journals from the convenience of a desktop computer. Improved database searching technology has made possible a number of complex approaches to searching, including: cross-disciplinary and multi-disciplinary sharing of information; tracking cited references and related references (papers with citations in common); and the ability to combine topics in a single search.

Computer searching requires the user to first consider all the databases in which pertinent information may reside. He will want to prioritize a list of the principal databases to search for a comprehensive identification of potentially relevant citations. The use of synonyms or variant word spellings becomes more important when approaching a computer search, as not all computer systems map or guide the user to all the relevant references. A mapped system would locate references indexed under *breast neoplasms* when the user entered *breast cancer,* whereas a system without mapping would not do so. The practitioner engaging in research-based practice will want to consider the librarian as an important resource for help and guidance through the maze of computerized sources, methods, and access points.

HEALTH CARE DATABASES

There are many databases you could use in conducting your search, but the following are the ones most frequently used by practitioners. Information regarding how to access these and other databases via the Internet is provided in Appendix B.

Principal Databases

Database	Principal Subject Coverage
MEDLINE	Medicine
CINAHL	Nursing and Allied Health
HealthSTAR	Health Care Administration

MEDLINE

The MEDLINE database is widely recognized as the premier source for bibliographic and abstract coverage of biomedical literature and is available via CD ROM or via the Internet. MEDLINE encompasses information from these print indexes: Index Medicus, Index to Dental Literature, and International Nursing Index. More than 3800 journals are indexed (National Library of Medicine [NLM], 1998). Although MEDLINE includes a nursing index, CINAHL is recognized as more comprehensive for the nursing discipline.

MEDLINE includes indexing in the following areas:

Allied health	Information science
Biological sciences	Physical sciences
Communication disorders	Population biology
Humanities	Reproductive biology

Coverage from 1966 to the present: 9 million records.

CINAHL

The CINAHL (Cumulative Index to Nursing and Allied Health Literature) database provides authoritative coverage of the literature related to nursing and the allied health disciplines (CINAHL Information Systems, 1998). Virtually all English language nursing publications (more than 1000 journals) are indexed along with publications of the American Nurses Association and the National League for Nursing. Primary journals from the following allied health fields are included:

Cardiopulmonary technology	Physical therapy
Emergency services	Physician assistant
Health education	Radiologic technology
Medical laboratory	Technology therapy
Medical assistants	Social service, health care
Medical records	Surgical technology
Occupational therapy	

CINAHL also selectively indexes materials in the following disciplines:

Alternative/complementary therapies	Consumer health
Biomedicine	Health science librarianship

In addition to journals, CINAHL selectively indexes materials using the following formats:

Audiovisual materials	Educational software
Conference proceedings	Health care books
Dissertations	Standards of professional practice

Coverage from 1982 to the present: 350,000 records.

HealthSTAR

HealthSTAR indexes published literature on health services, technology, administration, and research. It focuses on both the clinical and nonclinical aspects of health care delivery. Information in HealthSTAR is derived from MEDLINE, the Hospital Literature Index published by the American Hospital Association, and selected journals (National Library of Medicine, 1998). The following topics are included:

Accreditation	Health services research
Administration and planning of health facilities	Health insurance
	Laws and regulations
Effectiveness of procedures, programs, products, services, and processes	Licensure
	Personnel administration
Evaluation of patient outcomes	Quality assurance
Health policy	Services and manpower

In addition to journals, HealthSTAR selectively indexes materials using the following formats:

Books	Newspaper articles
Book chapters	Technical reports
Government documents	Theses
Meeting abstracts and papers	

Coverage from 1975 to the present: 3 million records.

Other Relevant Databases

A selected list of databases is provided below. Ask your librarian about local access to them if they are not available to you via the Internet.

Database	Principal Subject Coverage
PsycINFO	Psychology
Social Science Citation Index	Social Sciences
EMBASE	European-based Medicine
ERIC	Education
BIOETHICSLINE	Biomedical Ethics
CANCERLIT	Cancer
AIDSLINE	AIDS and HIV
The Cochrane Library	Systematic reviews of health care research

PsycINFO

PsycINFO indexes psychologically relevant material, including journal articles, dissertations, reports, book chapters, books, and other documents. Covered literature includes material from over 45 countries and written in more than 30 languages. Unrivaled in its depth of psychological coverage and respected worldwide for its high quality, the database selectively indexes materials from the fields of education, business, medicine, nursing, law, and social work (American Psychological Association, 1998).

Coverage from 1967 to the present: 1 million records.

Social SciSearch

Social SciSearch is a multi-disciplinary database covering the journal literature of the social sciences. It indexes 1700 journals spanning 50 disciplines, as well as covering selected items from over 3300 of the world's leading scientific and technical journals. Social SciSearch offers cited reference searching in addition to traditional searching by author and keyword (Institute for Scientific Information, 1998).

Coverage from 1972 to present: over 2.5 million records.

SciSearch

SciSearch is a multi-disciplinary science database covering the journal literature of the sciences. It indexes 5300 journals spanning over 158 disciplines.
SciSearch offers cited reference searching in addition to traditional searching by author and keyword (Institute for Scientific Information, 1998).
    Coverage from 1974 to present: over 7.5 million records.

EMBASE

EMBASE features comprehensive coverage of drugs and toxicology, clinical
medicine, basic biological sciences, biotechnology, bioengineering and bio-
physics, health affairs, pharmacy and pharmacoeconomics, psychiatry, environment and pollution, and forensic medicine. Selective coverage of the
following topics is also provided: nursing, dentistry, veterinary medicine,
normal psychology, and alternative medicine. Consider this database after
searching MEDLINE and CINAHL (Elsevier Science, 1998).
    Coverage from 1974 to present: over 6.5 million records.

ERIC

The Educational Resources Information Center (ERIC) is a U.S. federally
funded, nationwide information network designed to provide ready access
to education literature. It is the largest education database in the world,
containing journal articles, research reports, curriculum and teaching
guides, conference papers, and books (Educational Resources Information
Center, 1998).
    Coverage from 1966 to present: 900,000 records.

BIOETHICSLINE

BIOETHICSLINE is concerned with ethics and related public policy issues
in health care and biomedical research. Produced by the Kennedy Institute
of Ethics at Georgetown University, citations are derived from the literature
of law, medicine, the social sciences, philosophy, and the popular media
(National Library of Medicine, 1998).
    Coverage from 1973 to present: over 53,000 records.

CANCERLIT

CANCERLIT indexes cancer literature including journal articles, government reports, technical reports, meeting abstracts and papers, monographs,

letters, and theses. Comprehensive and international in scope, CANCERLIT is produced by the U.S. National Cancer Institute in cooperation with the National Library of Medicine (National Cancer Institute, 1998).

Coverage from 1976 to present: 1.4 million records.

AIDSLINE

AIDSLINE contains references to the published literature on HIV infections and acquired immune deficiency syndrome. It focuses on the biomedical, epidemiological, health care administration, oncologic, social, and behavioral sciences literatures. The file contain citations to journal articles, monographs, meeting abstracts and papers, newsletters, government reports, theses, and newspaper articles (National Library of Medicine, 1998).

Coverage from 1980 to present: over 140,000 records.

The Cochrane Library

The Cochrane Library is a regularly updated electronic library designed to make available the evidence needed to make informed health care decisions. The program presents the growing body of work of the Cochrane Collaboration and others interested in evidence-based medicine. Currently the library maintains four databases (Cochrane, 1998):

1. The Cochrane Database of Systematic Review
2. The Database of Abstracts of Reviews of Effectiveness
3. The Cochrane Controlled Trials Register
4. The Cochrane Review Methodology Database.

DATABASE SEARCHING STRATEGIES

Novice database searchers have a tendency to enter a search term in the form that is most familiar to them in their clinical setting. In most search systems, depending on the actual term used, this approach will result in the retrieval of documents but may not produce a comprehensive retrieval of relevant documents. If the term entered appeared in the title or abstract of a document, that document would certainly be retrieved. However, this approach could overlook documents that deal entirely with the topic of interest but do not use that particular term in the title or the abstract. Another disadvantage of a simple one-word search is that it may retrieve a large number of references that will be irrelevant to the clinical question.

The indexing systems of the databases are designed to help you focus your search and comprehensively retrieve references that are highly likely to be relevant to the specific aspect of a topic. To do this, you need to learn a few methods to take advantage of the databases' functions and indexing structure. The following sections will describe how to construct multistep searches that approach a topic from several directions and fully utilize the search capabilities of the database.

Using Keywords

Database search systems find relevant documents by searching for the entered terms in the title or abstract *and* by searching for documents that were indexed as relevant to that term. Most databases use controlled vocabulary, or keywords, to index the literature, meaning that each document is assigned terms from a predetermined vocabulary or list of terms. Although some online systems are beginning to offer automatic "mapping" to get you to the full range of system terms even though you have entered a nonsystem term, it is advisable to use the thesaurus for the specific database to learn what terms the system prefers.

If you enter the term "dysphagia," the system with mapping capability will automatically search for all documents indexed using the system term "deglutition disorders." In general, it is best to search using the more commonly used clinical term, in addition to the controlled vocabulary that approximates it. The two approaches will not retrieve identical lists of documents, and a combination of the two approaches will produce a more comprehensive search.

Making Your Search More Specific

Using Limits. MEDLINE and HealthSTAR both use *Medical Subject Headings* or MeSH vocabulary in their thesauri (NLM, 1998), whereas CINAHL employs the vocabulary found in the Nursing and Allied Health Subject Heading List, which offers a nursing-focused approach and terms (CINAHL Information Systems, 1998). When a document is entered into MEDLINE, CINAHL, or HealthSTAR, the entire document is assigned at least one major focus term from the database's official vocabulary by a team of experts; the major focus term reflects the major thrust of the document. When searching, the user can specify that the keywords entered express the major focus of the records to be retrieved. Executing a command to "limit to major focus" as a second step in a search will retrieve fewer documents than just entering the keywords themselves because documents that were indexed with the keyword as a minor focus will not be retrieved. There are times when you want the more inclusive retrieval and times when you want to be more selective.

Keywords that are quite broad often have subheadings, which are specific aspects of the keyword. Frequently used subheadings are etiology, therapy, diet therapy, complications, prevention, diagnosis, nursing, and rehabilitation. Using both a major focus term and one or more subheadings in your search can make your search more specific and avoid retrieval of irrelevant documents. It is worth finding out how the database system you are using presents subheadings under a particular keyword. The following search indicates the use of MeSH headings and limits.

Step	Enter	Nos. of Records Retrieved
1	deglutition disorders	6121
2	limit to major focus	3142
3	limit to subheadings rehabilitation, therapy	157

This search could be further narrowed using strategies discussed in the following paragraphs.

Using the Tree Structure. The CINAHL, MEDLINE, and HealthSTAR databases organize their keywords in a complex hierarchy, or tree structure, branching from broader terms to more specific ones. If you browse this tree structure, you will find that the general term "intestinal neoplasms" contains the branch "rectal neoplasms." Browsing the tree structure will inform you of all the more specific terms under the broader term (Lowe and Barnett, 1994), and thus enable you to select the specific term that is of interest. For example, under health behavior in the MEDLINE tree structure are three more specific terms: patient compliance, self-examination, and treatment refusal.

The tree structure can be used to either narrow or broaden your search. Some systems (e.g., PubMed) automatically "explode" a term, meaning that all documents indexed using more specific terms under the main term will be retrieved, whereas other systems require that you execute the "explode term" command to retrieve these documents. When you want to retrieve documents germane to both the general term and its more specific terms, it is advantageous to have the explode feature operating, whereas when you are interested only in the more general term, you will want to either turn the explode command off or not use it.

Boolean Operators. Boolean operators are system terms one incorporates into a search phrase to either narrow or broaden the search; *and, or,* and *not* are the most useful ones. Use *and* to retrieve records that include both keywords; for example, "computers and nursing" would retrieve only records pertinent to both nursing and computers. Use *or* to retrieve records with either of two keywords; the search phrase "AIDS *or* HIV" would retrieve records pertinent to either AIDS or HIV but need not address both in the same record. Use *not* to retrieve records with one keyword, but not another; "cancer not tumor" would retrieve records about cancer but would exclude those about tumors. The following is an example of how Boolean operators can be used to refine a search:

Step	Enter	Nos. of Records Retrieved
1	home health care	3436
2	HIV *or* AIDS	4765
3	1 *and* 2	72
4	long term care	3543
5	3 *not* 4	65

Methodological Filters. Computer literature searches can be focused to a specific type of report, which characterizes the nature of the information that constitutes the document or the manner in which it is conveyed (NLM, 1998). MEDLINE and CINAHL refer to these categories as "publication types." The following is a partial list of the publication types from those databases (see their thesauri for complete lists).

MEDLINE	CINAHL
clinical trial	clinical innovations
clinical trial, phase I	clinical trial
clinical trial, phase II	critical path
clinical trial, phase III	practice guidelines
clinical trial, phase IV	protocol
controlled clinical trial	questionnaire
guideline	research
meta-analysis	research instrument
practice guideline	review
randomized controlled trial	sensitivity and specificity
review literature	statistics
scientific integrity review	systematic review
technical report	

Note how the following use of a limit on publication types immediately zeroed in on state-of-the science summaries.

Step	Enter	No. of References Retrieved
1	Resuscitation, cardiopulmonary	693
2	limit to meta-analysis	4

Other Strategies. Assume a practitioner is interested in research on counseling women regarding the implications of having breast cancer and knows how to use keywords, Boolean operators, and subheadings. Notice how this search started broad and then added limits to access only highly relevant references.

Step	Enter	No. of References Retrieved
1	breast neoplasms	2174
2	limit to prevention, nursing psychosocial, education, familial, and genetic	876
3	limit to English language, adults ages 19–44, years 1990–present	237
4	limit to review articles	11

You need to be aware that retrieval using specific limits depends heavily on the quality of the indexing performed in the databases. If the indexing on a particular limit has been introduced recently, you will receive a false low return of references. For example, the term acquired immune deficiency was not a keyword in MEDLINE until 1983, which was several years after it was being discussed in the literature; thus, a search using the term will not retrieve documents on the topic prior to 1983. In addition, if a document has been added recently to the database, it may not yet have been assigned system indexing terms (e.g., MeSH terms); for this reason you should use common clinical terms as well as system keywords in your search.

Expanding Your Search

If your first search does not retrieve any references or retrieves very few, you will need to broaden your search. The tools to consider include employing synonyms or alternate keywords, the use of wildcard searching, and considering other databases or the use of the reference lists of highly relevant articles to identify other studies.

Synonyms and Alternative Keywords. Be flexible in the words you use to think about your topic, and conduct searches using a variety of terms and combinations of terms. To identify broader or alternative headings, consult the keywords list or the online thesaurus for the particular database, and rebuild the search applying newly identified keywords. The following list of searches, which was aimed at finding out about burns associated with automobile air bag deployment, shows the difference in retrieval when various terms and combinations of terms are employed.

Search	Terms	No. of References Retrieved
1	"air bags" and trauma	134
2	"air bag" and injuries	137
3	"air bag deployment" and injury	34
4	"air bags" and "eye injuries"	24
5	"air bags" and burns	11
6	"air bags" and "chemical burns"	5
7	"air bags" and "burn injury"	1
8	"air bag deployment" and "chemical burns"	0

Many of the documents retrieved in each search are duplicates of those retrieved by the other searches, but some documents will not be duplicates. Note that in these searches quotation marks were used to retrieve only documents in which two words occur together (i.e., you don't want all documents in which the term air occurs separate from bag). Whether you enter singular or plural terms can also make a difference in some cases (e.g., injury versus injuries). In summary, if you want comprehensive retrieval of studies, you will have to conduct a series of searches using different terms, different combinations of terms, and in some cases different limits.

Truncation or Wildcard Searching. Often there are a number of variations in the way a term is used, and you may want to identify references using all of them. Consider using the technique know as wildcard or truncation searching, which searches for variant spelled words, or more commonly, variant ending words. Common commands for wildcard searching include the asterisk (*) or dollar sign ($) at the point where the word may vary. Thus, nurs* retrieves: nurse, nursing, nurses, nursery. An interesting problem associated with this particular command is that it would retrieve references about infant breast feeding (nursing) as well as the profession of nursing.

Other Databases. If the techniques just described do not yield the kind of retrieval of references you are expecting, consider using an alternative database. Instead of using MEDLINE, maybe you should consider a more focused database such AIDSLINE, CANCERLIT, or BIOETHICSLINE. Consult the list provided earlier or ask your health science librarian for alternatives.

Reference Lists and Cited References. The reference lists or bibliographies of highly relevant articles can lead you to additional relevant older studies, both primary sources of information and other articles that were missed in the computer search. An additional strategy is to construct a cited reference search of these same highly relevant articles to find later studies that have included them in their bibliographies. Using computer databases such as Social SciSearch or SciSearch, you can identify authors citing a particular article from an earlier publication.

For example, a cited reference search was performed on a study published in the journal of *Pediatrics* in 1992. Among the articles that subsequently cited the study are four recent articles.

Original article:

Cronenwett, L., Stuckel, T., Kearney, M., Barrett, J., Covington, C., DelMonte, K., Reinhardt, R., and Rippe, L. (1992). Single daily bottle use in the early weeks postpartum and breast-feeding outcomes. *Pediatrics, 90:*760–766.

Citing articles:

Kuehl, J. (1997). Cup feeding the newborn: What you should know. *Journal of Perinatology and Neonatology Nursing, 11:*56–60.

Chezem, J., Montgomery, P., and Fortman, T. (1997). Maternal feelings after cessation of breast-feeding: Influence of factors related to employment and duration. *Journal of Perinatology and Neonatology Nursing, 11:*61–70.

Schubiger, G., Schwarz, U., and Tonz, O. (1997). UNICEF/WHO baby-friendly hospital initiative: Does the use of bottles and pacifiers in the neonatal nursery prevent successful breast-feeding? *European Journal of Pediatrics, 156:*874–877.

Hill, P.D., Humenick, S.S., Brennan, M.L., et al. (1997). Does early supplementation affect long-term breast-feeding? *Clinical Pediatrics, 36:*345–350.

Other Resources. If after searching the databases you still have identified very few studies relevant to your clinical question, you should not just conclude that no research has been done. Research might have been done but was not published or is just in the process of being published, or research might be under way relative to your question. Often it is useful to contact a researcher who has already published a report on the topic to determine if she has any other ongoing research or can direct you to unpublished papers or other research in progress. In the field of nursing, the Registry of Nursing Research, which is maintained by the Virginia Henderson International Nursing Library, contains biographical data about nurse researchers, their research programs, and summaries of their studies and their findings. This registry is available online to members of Sigma Theta Tau International (Sigma Theta Tau International, 1998). Other disciplines presumably have, or will be developing, similar registries.

The Internet. The Internet, particularly the World Wide Web, has brought a new dimension to searching for studies, people, and other information on a wide range of topics. The experienced Internet searcher knows it should be viewed with both delight and concern as a medical information tool (Silberg, Lundberg, and Musacchio, 1997). Resources on the Internet vary widely in terms of accuracy—just because information is on the Internet does not mean it is valid or verifiable. Specific information regarding the addresses of online databases and other electronic resources is provided in Appendix B.

The home page of the National Institutes of Health (http://nih.gov/) will link you to a variety of other resources, such as the sites of the 24 separate institutes and centers within the National Institutes of Health (NIH). Through this site you also can access the CRISP system, which is a database containing information about the research ventures supported by the United States Public Health Service. Links to lists of funded grants can also be obtained through the home pages of the Agency for Health Care Policy and Research (http://www.ahcpr.gov:80/) and the National Institute for Nursing Research (http://www.nih.gov/ninr/).

Another approach would be to locate a listserv through which discussions on the topic of interest to you take place via electronic mail (e-mail). There is a specific, but very easy, procedure for signing onto a listserv, and then you will receive the automatically distributed messages members of the list contribute. The dialog is often informative, and you can ask a question of all persons on the list just by sending an e-mail message to the designated address. Examples of Web sites for listservs are as follows:

> http://www.springnet.com/np/nplstsrv.htm), for advanced practice nurses
> http://www.auhs.edu/library/resource/pt-lists.htm), for physical therapists
> http://www.call24-med.com/linksot.htm), for occupational therapists.

RETRIEVING REPORTS

You may need to rely on several avenues to actually retrieve pertinent study reports that are not available in the local library. Your local librarians undoubtedly will help you initiate an interlibrary loan request, which usually involves completing a request form. Be sure to have complete information on the articles and books you request; many of the databases assign an accession number to each reference, and you may be asked to include this on your request. If you are a guest user of a library and thus not eligible for the library's interlibrary loan service, the staff may advise you of alternative resources, such as a state library or loaning network. Interlibrary loans often take several weeks, and there may be a charge.

If you use the Internet PubMed site of the National Library of Medicine to search MEDLINE, there is an option of ordering an article of interest as part of each article's page. The service is called Loansome Doc, and details regarding setting up an account are available when you indicate you want to order an article.

U.S. Government documents are available at selected academic and public libraries which agree to provide access to all members of the public. Increasingly, government documents are being made available over the Internet (see Appendix B). Databases of dissertations and other special reports are usually not available in small libraries, necessitating a search of library catalogs to determine what is available; once identified in the catalog, many of these documents are not available from the university where they are located—instead they must be purchased from an organization such as UMI, a for-profit company that archives over 1.4 million dissertations, theses, books, periodicals, newspapers, and scholarly collections. Response is typically rapid (see entry in Appendix B).

SUMMARY

This chapter has covered a broad spectrum of strategies and specific guidance for locating studies and state-of-the-science summaries that may be relevant to the clinical question you want to answer using research evidence. Because your practice is within a particular clinical area, you do not have to be familiar with all the databases described in this chapter. Rather, there will be two or three that you will use regularly, and hence, you will become familiar with their terms, indexing structure, and searching commands.

Searching for relevant studies requires that you be a detective of sorts. To be successful, you will need to track down leads from a variety of sources and be sensitive to the language clues embedded in your leads and consider incorporating them into your search. One student who was searching for studies related to the accuracy with which the elderly take their medications noted that the term "polypharmacy" was used in an abstract. The term was unknown to her but when she became aware of its meaning and relevance to her search and incorporated it into her search, a whole new array of documents were retrieved that weren't available when she just entered "elderly" and "medication adherence."

Many search systems have a great deal of guidance incorporated into them to help you find what you are interested in and to actually teach you to become a better searcher. Considerable information about the language of the database can be found in the thesaurus of the browser, and the actual use of the system's functions is described in a tutorial or HELP section. Other systems prompt you or make suggestions of alternative terms or search strategies as you conduct your search. These search systems are becoming increasingly user-friendly and can actually be fun to use. More important, they make finding potentially relevant studies an efficient, informative, and speedy step of research-based practice.

References

American Psychological Association (1998). PsycINFO-Information Services in Psychology. Online site: http://www.apa.org/psycinfo/

CINAHL Information Systems (1998). *Cumulative Index to Nursing and Allied Health (CINAHL).* Online site: http://www.cinahl.com

Cochrane Library (1998). Online site: http://www.cochrane.co.uk/

Dumas, M.A., Shurpin, K., and Gallo, K. (1995). Search and research: Getting started in clinical research. *Journal of the American Academy of Nurse Practitioners, 7*:591–597.

Educational/Resources Information Center (1998). Online site: http://ericir.syr.edu/eric

Elsevier Science (1998). EMBASE. Online site: http://www.elsevier.com/

Index Medicus (1879). *Index Medicus: A Quarterly Classified Record of the Current Medical Literature of the World.* New York: Leypoldt.

Institute for Scientific Information (1998). Online site: http://www.isinet.com/

Joos, I., Whitman, N.I., Smith, M.J., and Nelson, R. (1992). *Computers in Small Bytes: The Computer Workbook.* New York: NLN Press.

Lowe, H.J., and Barnett, G.O. (1994). Understanding and using the medical subject headings (MeSH) vocabulary to perform literature searches. *Journal of the American Medical Association, 271*:1103–1108.

National Cancer Institute (1998). CancerNet cancer information. Online site: http://cancernet.nci.nih.gov/

National Library of Medicine (1998). AIDSLINE. Online site: http://www.nlm.nih.gov/pubs/factsheets/aidsline.html

National Library of Medicine (1998). BIOETHICSLINE. Online site: http://www.nlm.nih.gov/pubs/factsheets/online_databases.html#bioethics

National Library of Medicine (1998). HealthSTAR. Online site: http://www.nlm.nih.gov/pubs/factsheets/healthstar.html

National Library of Medicine (1998). *Medical Subject Headings: Annotated Alphabetic List.* Bethesda, MD: National Library of Medicine.

National Library of Medicine (1998). MEDLINE. Online site: http://www.nlm.nih.gov/databases/medline.html

Sigma Theta Tau International, the International Honor Society of Nursing (1998). Virginia Henderson International Nursing Library. Online site: http://www.stti.iupui.edu/library/

Silberg, W.M., Lundberg, G., and Musacchio, R.A. (1997). Assessing, controlling, and assuring the quality of medical information on the Internet: Caveat Lector et Viewor—Let the reader and viewer beware. *Journal of the American Medical Association, 277*:1244–1245.

Ulrich's International Periodicals Directory (36th ed). (1997). New York: Bowker.

6

Reading Research Reports

Once you have a collection of possibly relevant research reports assembled, you will want to eliminate any studies that do not pertain to your clinical question. For example, if you were specifically interested in how seizures affect adults' functioning in their job in the hours after a seizure, you will want to eliminate those that address seizures in children, those that examine psychological issues of persons with seizures, and those that study long-term effects of seizures on family and social relationships. You may, however, want to keep the ones pertaining to how having seizures affects social functioning, because some may examine the effects of having seizure on job performance, including pre- and postdromal states. Sometimes, you can eliminate studies simply by reading the abstract, but you may need to examine the purpose statement of the study, usually found early in the report. You may even have to look deeper into the report to see if the study addresses the specific issue in which you have an interest (e.g., postdromal job performance) as one of many issues examined under a broader term (e.g., social functioning). The characteristics of the people who made up the sample and the setting in which the study was conducted should also be noted. With these pieces of information, you can decide if the research study addresses your question and is likely to be applicable to your setting; if it meets both criteria, it's worth investing your time to read and appraise in full.

SOURCES OF REPORTS

Research reports are tailored to the interests and background of the journal's readers, which influences the areas of emphasis in the report. Thus, you should note whether the journal or book in which the report is published is a research journal or a clinical journal; you should also note whether reports to the journal must undergo peer review, and whether the journal publishes reports predominately from one health care discipline or is truly multi-disciplinary.

Reports in research journals are often written primarily for other researchers and, consequently, have many details about the research methods and about the data analysis. If the research journal is peer-reviewed, there is a high likelihood that the report has been read by expert researchers in the field who have deemed it scientifically sound. Unfortunately, practitioners sometimes don't relate to studies in research journals because the questions examined seem unimportant, the report may involve complex statistics, and the report of the findings may lack sufficient detail to be of use to practitioners.

In contrast, research reports in clinical journals often address questions that are directly applicable to practice. They typically have short research methods and analysis sections and long discussion sections in which the ramifications for practice are addressed. Reports in clinical journals, even peer-reviewed journals, may or may not have been reviewed by expert researchers. This lack of a demanding quality screen may be further compounded by the abbreviated information presented about the methods of the study. Even though the results are reported in detail and their implications are considered, the reader is put in the position of having to trust that the methods used were sound.

Although the contrast between the two types of journals is not always as severe as just portrayed, the differentiation is important enough to keep in mind. Fortunately, many clinical journals are providing more information about how studies were conducted (sometimes in sidebars), so the reader can appraise the scientific soundness of studies, and some research journals have been created specifically to present research to practitioners, rather than to other researchers. These journals balance the presentation of information about methods with the discussion of practice implications in ways that are both readable and useful.

Identification of the disciplinary origins of the journal in which the report is published is relevant to appraisal because every discipline has a unique perspective on health and illness. These perspectives are like lenses through which the discipline sees reality, and they determine what the discipline sees as the main features of reality. Within the health care disciplines, the biomedical perspective has been dominant for years, but others have been used and are being articulated with greater clarity and persuasiveness. These views include psychosocial, cognitive, psychocognitive, behavioral, functional, humanistic, emancipatory, and holistic perspectives. When you are reading a study you should try to identify the philosophical perspective that is being used so that you can consider the findings within the context in which they were produced. Getting in touch with the perspectives of other disciplines, and even with the diversity of perspectives within one's own discipline or specialty, can be enlightening in that it can reveal ways of thinking about issues and problems that are fresh and enriching. A perspective may be quite different from the one you have chosen to use in everyday practice—it may be more holistic, based more in psychological behaviorism, or more traditionally biomedical. However, taking note of the perspective that shaped a study will enable you to determine the degree to which the findings will fit with how you view what you do. The findings of a study may persuade you to add a new dimension to your thinking about a clinical issue, or you may just remind yourself that the research was done from another disciplinary perspective.

STEPS IN THE APPRAISAL OF FINDINGS

You are now ready to start appraising the findings of a study—an overview of the steps involved is displayed in Box 6–1. Appraising involves (a) reading the research report for an understanding of the important components of the study and composing a synopsis, (b) appraising the findings

for scientific credibility, clinical significance, and applicability to your practice. In this chapter, issues related to the reading of research reports and to writing a synopsis of the study will be addressed. Issues related to appraising the findings will be addressed in Chapter 7.

READING INTERACTIVELY[1]

Reading research reports carefully and in their entirety is a prerequisite to appraisal—skimming or even quick reading them will not result in sufficient knowledge of the particulars to allow you to appraise them. You should know that it is often surprising, even to persons who read research reports on a regular basis, how long it takes to really acquire an understanding of how a study was conducted and what was found. It is not something most people can do quickly, although with practice you will get faster. It is tedious because most research reports are quite dense; that is, every sentence contains important information, so if you aren't paying full attention, you may gloss over information that you will need later. Fortunately, research reports are usually written in fairly standardized formats, which keep the reader oriented and make it easy to move around within the report.

If you are to come away from reading a research report with understanding of how the study was done and what was found, you will have to be an active reader. To read actively means that you monitor your thinking by noting whether you are understanding what you are reading, and if you aren't, you break out of reading to reread previous sections, dig into the tables where data is presented, or go to another source that will help fill in any gaps in your knowledge. You also need to go beyond understanding what is said to question what is said and what is not said. If participants' answers were scored, you want to be thinking: How were category labels or numbers assigned to answers? Did more than one person do the scoring? Was there any check on the extent to which the two scorers would produce the same or similar score if they were rating the same answer? This information is

---

[1]If you are quite accustomed to reading research reports, you may want to skip this section and go to the next section, Completing a Synopsis.

essential in deciding whether bias could have been introduced by the scoring decision. If the researcher did not provide this information, skepticism about the results enters your thinking during your reading of the report.

At first you may find it difficult just to get a sense of what the study's purpose was, how it was conducted, and what was found. As you get more comfortable with reading studies, you'll find yourself responding to what you read in a more evaluative manner. Although objective appraisal of a study requires that you eventually separate the facts regarding the study from your judgment of the study, your initial reading of a report will undoubtedly be a "messy" mixture of comprehending and reacting. You already have a preferred way of reading to acquire comprehension of materiel (e.g., use of a highlighter, marginal notes, a note sheet), and that's fine, but observe yourself to make sure that you are also reacting to what you read, not just pulling out the important points. Reactions include noting concerns regarding ways of doing the study that could have affected the results, omission of important information, and lack of logical connections between the stages of the research process.

An illustration of reacting would involve questioning the outcomes of a study in which an intervention was tested because you think they are not sensitive enough to the intervention. For example, in a study of the effects of a preoperative teaching intervention for the elderly, the intervention did not decrease the days of hospitalization after surgery as hypothesized. You may think that reducing the days of hospitalization was not an appropriate outcome to use in this study because the number of days of hospitalization is so heavily influenced by other factors, such as days of certification based on admitting diagnosis and availability of beds at the next level of care. Choice of an outcome that is not sensitive to an intervention, or that is more heavily influenced by other variables, may produce results indicating that the intervention had no effect—i.e., there was no difference in the outcomes of the treatment groups—when in fact it was the researcher's choice of outcome variables that determined this result. If another outcome, or outcomes, were studied, the findings may have shown that intervention made a difference. It is important to respect reactions of these kinds that you may have to a study, because as a clinician you may have insights into the dynamics of a situation not considered by the researcher, and the factors you identify may have influenced the results of the study. Your most basic goal in reading is to understand, but at the same time you want to be challenging how the study was conceived, how it was done, what types of patients were studied, how the data was interpreted, and why the results may have come out as they did.

Assumptions

Noticing what is not said in a report is also important. Assumptions on which the study rests often are not explicitly stated because the researcher is unaware of them, yet they can affect all aspects of the study. A study of how people deal with dyspnea may be based implicitly on the notion that dyspnea is a symptom that must be controlled, in contrast to viewing it as a sensory experience accompanied by a cognitive interpretation, emotional response, and coping behavior (Steele and Shaver, 1992). The assumption that dyspnea is a symptom that must be controlled will affect the questions that are asked about dyspnea as well as how it is studied and measured. Biological and physiological views of human health and illness are still subtly dominant in health care research, and can lead to ways of studying issues that aren't consistent with more holistic perspectives. A study can be well designed and well conducted, but if you don't accept its assumptions, you will question the credibility of its findings.

Limits of Reports

A research report is really a summary of the what, why, and how of a study as well as a reporting of its data-based knowledge claims. As a summary, it contains what the researcher thought were the most important particulars a reader needs to know to understand what was done and what was found, but you will inevitably find that you are missing pieces of information that you think have bearing on the results and conclusions. For example, in a study about the relationship between physical health and depression among older adults, you may find that the researcher did not provide you with sufficient information about whether the person's social network had changed in the last year, and you are left wondering whether the death of peers could have contributed to the presence, absence, or level of depression.

Second, you may find that the report lacks certain methodological details necessary for full appraisal. When faced with omissions in the report, you have two choices: (1) live with it as a limit of published communication, or (2) contact the researcher and ask your question. E-mail is a minimally intrusive, quick, low-cost way of making contact. In most cases the researcher's answer will either reassure you that the issue was taken into account or reinforce your initial reaction that it was an uncontrolled variable at work in the study. Either way, you will feel better about your appraisal because it will be based on more complete information.

Formats

Formats of research reports vary somewhat from journal to journal, but most follow the logic of the research process. This consistency of format will keep you oriented as you read a report and will help you locate particular items in a report that you may have overlooked on first reading. All journals use headings and subheadings to label the various sections of the report, but the subheadings vary, as does the content included in each section. A typical format is displayed in Box 6–2.

Abstract. Some journals include 100- to 200-word abstracts which summarize the entire report immediately after the title of the research reports; others do not. Often you will be able to tell just from the abstract whether the study is relevant to your clinical question.

Introduction. Perhaps the biggest difference in formats is in how previous knowledge about the subject is dealt with, the most common approach being to present background information and a review of prior research in the untitled introduction that opens the report. Background information can include data supporting the significance or prevalence of a problem, explanatory models that have been developed and tested, or a clinical rationale for doing the study. The amount of background information presented varies, depending on the journal, the author, and the state of knowledge about the issue; and an explanatory model, or theoretical framework, may or may not be specified in the introduction. Findings produced within the context of a particular model serve to test and further develop the model. In reverse, the model serves to link the findings to other knowledge on the topic by locating them within a larger framework. The findings of studies conducted without a conceptual or theoretical model are at risk of being isolated tidbits which are difficult to weave together with other knowledge about the issue. Knowledge about an issue is built piece by piece, study by study, finding by finding, and as a result, at some point a cohesive and comprehensive model is needed to explain how findings fit into the larger picture.

Almost all introductions include some kind of review of research already conducted relevant to the topic. Some reviews of prior research are summative and provide a useful overview of research in the area with comments regarding the most consistent findings, the studies that don't fit the trend, what issues have received little attention, and what knowledge is still in question. Other reviews of prior research are more selective in that they present the findings of four or five important studies in the area, but refrain from commentary.

In addition to background information and previous findings, most introductions also include an explicit statement of purpose or of the research objectives. Other times the purposes take the form of a list of hypotheses the study will test, or a statement of the research question,

---

Box 6–2

Typical Research Report Format

- Abstract
- Introduction
  Background
  Review of prior studies
  Statement of purpose
- Methods
  Sample/participants
  Measures
  Procedure
- Results
- Discussion
- References

e.g., "This study seeks to uncover the social processes that lead a person in a program for addicts to view himself or herself as capable of abstinence from substances."

Methods. The methodology of the study may be presented under one heading or broken down under several subheadings. Sometimes this section starts out with either a declaration of the research design used in the study, e.g., "This cross-sectional study was conducted. . . ." Other times the study design is not explicitly identified. Usually there is a section or paragraph describing how the sample was constituted, and the setting in which the study was conducted. Descriptions of the participants may be presented in the methods section or in the results section using a combination of descriptive statistics, narrative description, and/or statistical tests comparing the groups at the beginning of the study.

Ideally, the variables being studied are defined by a combination of conceptual definitions and the measures used to stand in for each concept, i.e., the operational definition. If measures were used, there usually is a discussion of what the measure evaluates, what it consists of, how it was administered, and what previous experiences have been with that measure, that is, its reliability and validity performance in the past. If the study involved an intervention, there should be a detailed description of how the intervention was delivered and whether any checks were done to ensure that it was consistently delivered.

The procedure subsection usually describes the sequence of research actions involved in collecting the data, including how participants were recruited, how instruments were calibrated or set up, how laboratory tests were performed, how interviews or observations were conducted, and how coding was done. Data analysis techniques are also addressed in the methods section, sometimes under a subheading, sometimes not. If the study was a qualitative study, the analytical technique used to find patterns, meaning, and themes in the data will be described. For quantitative studies, the statistical analyses and any adjustments to the data that were performed will be described.

Results. Report sections are often organized by grouping the findings according to the research questions or the hypotheses. This organization of the results is usually very helpful to the reader. In quantitative studies descriptive statistics are usually reported first followed by inferential statistics. Once data related to the main questions of the study have been presented, data related to subgroups will be presented. The results should include sufficient detail for you to get a sense of how groups compared, how variables were associated, and how likely a particular research hypothesis is to be true. In addition to narrative reporting, some combination of tables, charts, diagrams, and statistics is often provided. There is an expectation in scientific reporting that the results section present summarized data with as little interpretation as possible. The exception to this is qualitative research, which by nature involves intertwined data acquisition and data interpretation. Qualitative studies should provide you with a sense of how the researcher moved from raw data (e.g., quotes or observations) to identification of social or psychological processes or categories.

Discussion. In the discussion (also called conclusion) section the researcher should offer an interpretation of what the results mean. There should be a strong linkage between the results and the researcher's conclusions. The first part of this discussion should pertain directly to the research questions and the data, but may also include some speculation regarding why the findings are as they are. The researcher should connect the findings of the current study to previous findings by discussing similarities and possible reasons for differences. In later parts of the discussion the researcher may extend the interpretation beyond the conditions of the study and its findings. When extending, the researcher may also surmise regarding what implications the results have for future research, for theory development in the domain, for clinical practice, or for professional education.

References. References consist of a list of sources cited in the report. In addition to the documentation of sources of information, they can be invaluable to the reader who is interested in locating additional information regarding a specific population, setting, measure, or outcome.

COMPLETING A SYNOPSIS

After having the read the report thoroughly, it will be valuable to immediately complete a written synopsis of the study using the synopsis questions that will be provided. The synopsis of how the study was done and what was found will serve several purposes: (a) as a check on whether you have an adequate grasp of the study's elements; (b) as an extraction of the essential information that will be needed to appraise the findings and their applicability; and (c) as a way of retaining the essential information that will be necessary if you will be appraising findings across several studies. The synopsis mainly involves a recording of the essential elements of the study, and does not involve judging the study—this will be done in the appraisal. If you have carefully read the report and understood what was done and found, completing the synopsis will be straightforward and require little time. If you are new to reading research reports, however, you may find yourself having to look back into the report several times in order to complete the synopsis questions.

SUMMARY

Recognizing and becoming familiar with the formats used to report information is the first step in becoming comfortable with research reports and in acquiring facility in using the information contained therein. Research reports are in essence a genre of literature that has stylistic features that serve its purposes. Once you've spent some time reading in this genre, you'll find they really aren't as impenetrable as they first seem. This is particularly true as you read within a particular topical area and become familiar with its specialized language, the variables that are of interest, the research methods used, and the theoretical models that bind findings together into a coherent explanation of how things work in a particular domain of health care knowledge.

Reference

Steele, B., and Shaver, J. (1992). The dyspnea experience: Nociceptive properties and a model for research and practice. *Advances in Nursing Science, 15*:64–76.

Broad Issues in
the Appraisal
of Findings

Before proceeding to specific questions for appraising the findings of a single research study, the broad issues underlying appraisal need to be addressed. These broad issues are fundamental building blocks that must be understood to correctly and fully benefit from the questions provided for single-study appraisal, as well as those for appraisal of collective evidence and of a state-of-the-science summary.

This chapter contains what is probably the most abstract content in the book. There are many technical terms and explanations of research concepts, which makes it quite different in tone and density from the preceding chapters. The chapter starts out with an explanation of why five sets of questions are provided for appraisal of findings of single studies rather than a single set. Then the appraisal areas of synopsis, credibility, clinical significance, and applicability are each described in considerable detail. The discussion of credibility examines several forms of the term "validity" and how they relate to the appraisal approach used in this book. The chapter ends with a detailed explanation of the measures of clinical significance which will be used extensively in subsequent chapters.

APPRAISING FINDINGS, NOT STUDIES

Unlike critiques you may have done in the past, when seeking research-based answers for clinical questions it is the findings that are appraised, not the study per se—the findings are the knowledge product you are considering using. You will be required to pass judgment on the design and conduct of the study, but you will be doing so because their quality affects whether or not you consider the findings to be credible. The clinical significance and the applicability of the findings are also determined by the methods of the study, albeit more on *how* the study was designed than on *how well* it was designed.

Most often you will be interested in several or all of the findings of a study, but there will be times when, because of your clinical question, you will be interested in just one of the findings. There may also be occasions when you judge one of the findings of a study to be credible but another finding of that same study to be lacking in credibility. This would occur, for instance, when the study design did not control an extraneous variable and you think that variable could have influenced one of the outcome variables but not another. In still another scenario, you may be interested in several findings and decide that all of them are credible, but you may appraise some as clinically significant and others as clinically insignificant. Any of these situations would require you to think separately about the individual findings from a study rather than think about them as a group.

Throughout the discussions of appraisal and in the appraisal questions provided, there will be reference to "findings." However, you will have to decide whether you are considering a singular finding or the group of findings from a study. And you will have to be prepared for the likelihood that there will be times when you start out appraising "the findings" as a group but have to switch to appraising the individual findings of a study separately. Regrettably, appraisal of individual findings makes the appraisal process more complicated, but the complexity is inherent in the reality that most research studies produce more than one knowledge claim, and each should be appraised on its own merits.

FIVE SETS OF APPRAISAL QUESTIONS

Clinical health care studies examine a wide array of questions using many different research designs. When a body of research literature consists of studies using diverse designs, appraising the findings is demanding because knowledge of the unique features of each type of design is required. Appraisal guides for single studies achieve the greatest discernment when the questions provided are specific to the methodological standards unique to each type of study design. For this reason five sets of questions for appraising the findings of single studies have been developed as the basis for the approach used in this book—one for each of the five most commonly used research designs.

The five research designs and the clinical topics most commonly associated with each design are displayed in Table 7–1. The research design of the

Table 7–1. **Combinations of Research Designs and Associated Clinical Topics**

Research Design	Clinical Topics
Non-experimental, qualitative methods	Patient experiences with health and illness or social processes associated with health and illness
Non-experimental, descriptive methods (including survey)	Patient experiences or factors affecting health, illness, and health-related responses
Non-experimental, correlational methods	Patient experiences or factors affecting health, illness, and health-related responses
Experimental methods	Interventions, therapies, preventive services
Quasi-experimental methods	Interventions, therapies, preventive services

study under consideration will be the basis for choosing the appropriate set of questions for the findings of a single study; later the clinical topics will serve as the basis for choosing the appropriate set of questions when appraising collective evidence from several or many studies (addressed in Chapter 9). At this point it is advisable to look at the five sets of appraisal questions for single studies which are displayed in Appendix I; even though you will not be delving into these questions until Chapter 8, you should note how the four appraisal areas (i.e., synopsis, credibility, clinical significance, and applicability) recur in each of the five sets and how the questions in each appraisal area are specific to the particular research design.

Examples of Design Types

Study Using a Non-experimental Qualitative Methodology. Kearney, M.H., Murphy, S., Irwin, K., and Rosenbaum, M. (1995). Salvaging self: A grounded theory of pregnancy on crack cocaine. *Nursing Research, 44*:208–213.

Grounded theory methodology was used to develop a description of how pregnant crack cocaine users perceived their problems and responded to them. Comparative analysis of in-depth interviews with 60 pregnant or postpartum women who used crack cocaine on average at least once per week during pregnancy identified a threatened selfhood as the major problem and salvaging self as the basic social psychological process by which women attempted to redirect their lives. Actions included strategies of harm reduction and stigma management aimed at reducing damage to the fetus, their identities, and the maternal-child relationship.

Study Using a Non-experimental, Descriptive Survey Methodology. Valdini, A., and Cargill, L.C. (1997). Access and barriers to mammography in New England community health centers. *Journal of Family Practice, 45*:243–249.

A consecutive series of questionnaires were administered by staff of 32 community health centers in six New England states to low-income women over age 40 who attended the clinics; 2943 (95%) completed the questionnaire, which showed that 55% of the women aged 50 and older had mammography done during the last 2 years, whereas only 45% of the women aged 40–49 had. Most women who had not had a mammography said it was because they thought the test was not important. Expense and lack of insurance were secondary reasons.

Study Using a Non-experimental, Correlational Methodology. Badger, T.A. (1993). Physical health impairment and depression among older adults. *IMAGE: Journal of Nursing Scholarship, 25*:325–330.

Factors contributing to depression among a convenience sample of 80 independently living, older adults were examined. Persons with higher levels of physical health impairment experienced significantly more depression, and the two variables had a correlation of $r = .41$ ($p < .01$). In addition, persons with moderate to severe physical health impairment reported more problem drinking at a level that was statistically significant. The mediating variables of social resources, belief in one's ability to affect the important outcomes of one's life, and economic resources together explained 58% of the variance in depression.

Study Using a Randomized Experimental Methodology. Meydani, S.N., et al. (1997). Vitamin E supplementation and in vivo immune response in healthy elderly subjects. *Journal of American Medical Association, 277*:1380–1386.

A randomized, double-blind, placebo-controlled study of the effects of three dosage levels of vitamin E on six in vivo indexes of immune response were studied in 88 healthy, elderly adults. The 200-mg/d dosage group had several significant increases in cell-mediated immunity and antibody titers. No adverse effects were observed with vitamin E supplementation during the 235-day study.

Study Using a Quasi-Experimental Methodology. Pickler, R.H., Higgins, K.E., and Crummette, B.D. (1993). The effect of nonnutritive sucking on bottle-feeding stress in preterm infants. *Journal of Gynecology and Neonatal Nursing, 22*:230–234.

The effects of nonnutritive sucking on the physiological and behavioral stress reactions of 20 preterm infants during and after early bottle feeding were studied. The 10 infants who were provided nonnutritive sucking for five minutes before and after feeding were matched with 10 control infants. Infants who received nonnutritive sucking before and after bottle feedings were more likely to be in a quiescent behavior state five minutes after the feeding and had higher feeding performance scores than those in the control group.

Perceptions of Designs

Some researchers and research consumers view findings that are based on quantified data as more objective and reliable than findings arrived at via explicit interpretation and represented in words; hence, they view quantified findings as more "scientific." Others recognize that some assumption and interpretation exists in the conduct of all research, particularly when measuring, counting, and assigning numbers to real world entities and states; as a result, one form of data is not inherently "more scientific" than others. The position taken in this book is that some clinical entities lend themselves to being quantified, whereas others do not and are best captured using some combination of observation, interviewing, field notes, transcripts, categorization systems, or interpretive narratives.

There is more agreement that each research design has different strengths and different vulnerabilities to bias, confounding, error, or reduction of meaning. Generally, in evaluating the effectiveness of interventions, evidence from a randomized clinical trial is considered the "highest" form of evidence, and there are good reasons for holding randomized clinical trials in high regard for this purpose. Randomized clinical trials are less prone to error from initial differences between the groups being compared; however, not all important clinical questions can be studied via randomized clinical trials, and useful, valid information and understandings can be obtained using other research designs.

Although non-experimental designs and quasi-experimental designs lack sufficient controls to confirm cause-and-effect relationships, they are useful in discovering and initially verifying relationships between factors that may be important. Also, these designs are often able to capitalize on real-world situations providing unique opportunities to explore how personal and contextual factors affect what occurs. The meaning that experiences and events have for persons is often captured with the greatest richness by qualitative studies. Thus, each type of design serves functions that others may not, and there really is no one "best" design; rather, the best design is the one that will answer the research question and is feasible to conduct.

APPRAISAL AREAS

In appraising the findings of a single study, the features that must be taken into account are (a) how the study was conducted and what was found, (b) whether the findings are credible, (c) whether the findings are clinically significant, and (d) whether the findings can be safely and effectively applied in a specific situation. To appraise these features, each set of appraisal questions for a single study is divided into subsets called synopsis, credibility profile, clinical significance profile, and applicability profile. Together, these subset areas constitute a comprehensive and clinically meaningful appraisal format.

Appraisal Subset Areas
Synopsis
Credibility profile
Clinical significance profile
Applicability profile

Synopsis

In the previous chapter it was suggested that immediately after reading a report, you complete a synopsis using the questions provided in the synopsis subset. The essential elements of a study vary depending on the design of the study, hence a different subset of synopsis questions is provided in each of the five sets of appraisal questions for single studies. The written synopsis provides a sketch of how the study was conceptualized, designed, and conducted, and what the findings were. Completing the synopsis is really the preparatory work of appraisal in that it assembles the necessary informational pieces that will be required for the appraisal of credibility, clinical significance, and applicability.

Credibility

Credible findings are produced by studies that were conducted in scientifically sound ways. More specifically, credible findings are produced if the study was based on plausible logic and conducted in a way that took into account, or controlled, extraneous variables that could have influenced the findings. The credibility of the findings rests on the many aspects of the study's logic and design, including the methods by which participants were recruited and placed in groups, sample size, the conditions under which treatments were delivered, how data were collected, and the ways in which the data were analyzed. If each of these aspects was appropriate and sound, the researcher's account of the data is believed.

When appraising a study one has to go beyond taking note of the findings to consider whether there was anything about the way the study was conceived, designed, or carried out that may have distorted the portrayal of reality that the findings supply. If in conducting the appraisal you determine that the researcher allowed bias to enter the conduct of the study, allowed extraneous variables to influence the data, or reached erroneous statistical or thematic conclusions, you will decide that the picture of reality that the findings suggest is not a true representation of reality; that is, the findings are not credible. On the other hand, if you think bias and extraneous variables were well controlled and the researcher reached sound, data-based conclusions, you will judge the findings to be credible; i.e., you will view them as valid and trustworthy because they were produced by careful scientific methodology.

Variations on Validity

The matter of credibility is closely related to what others have called internal validity (Cook and Campbell, 1979; Krathwohl, 1985). There are actually several forms of "validity" that relate to research: internal validity, statistical conclusion validity, external validity, and construct validity. These variations can be confusing. Although the meaning of each of these terms will be explained, the appraisal methods used in this book will not use these terms per se; instead, the concepts will be incorporated into the appraisal questions using more clinical language.

Internal Validity. Internal validity, which is a major component of the term credibility as it is used in this book, refers to the trustworthiness of a study's findings. In appraising a study we must ask: Are the findings of this study valid? Do they faithfully and accurately portray real-world events, processes, cause and effect, or experience? To answer this question in the affirmative we must be confident that the conduct of the study as a whole was characterized by high internal validity, meaning that bias and unwanted influences, i.e., extraneous variables, were well controlled. An example of studies whose findings were challenged on the basis of low internal validity were early studies comparing care provided by nurse practitioners (NP) and certified nurse-midwives (CNM) to that provided by physicians. The findings rather consistently established that care provided by NPs and CNMs was of equivalent or superior quality to that provided by physicians, particularly in the areas of communication, preventive care, patient outcomes, and continuity (Brown and Grimes, 1993). However, the internal validity of these findings was questioned because many of the studies did not take into account (i.e., control) the possibility that patients treated by physicians are sicker or at higher risk for complications than NP or CNM patients. Thus, a confounding or extraneous variable influenced the findings. This was a legitimate criticism of some of these studies; however, in their meta-analysis of these studies Brown and Grimes used statistical methods to control for potential differences in client risk and still found equivalent or more favorable outcomes to be associated with NP or CNM care. The use of this "statistical control" in analyzing the results of these studies added considerable confidence to the collective conclusion of these studies that nurse-provided care compares favorably to physician-provided care with equivalent patients in similar settings.

There are many potential sources of unwanted influences, i.e., threats to internal validity, and research designs and protocols have been developed to control them; nevertheless, they may have affected the results unknowingly, which is of particular concern in studies examining cause and effect (Cook and Campbell, 1979). When we say that we have confidence in the internal validity of the findings of an intervention study, we are saying that we have confidence that the design and protocols of the study eliminated, controlled, or took into account all factors influencing the outcome variable other than the treatment variable; in so doing, the study truly evaluated the effects of the experimental treatment. Random assignment of participants to treatment groups and control over the conditions and procedures of a study are the best strategies for constraining unwanted sources of influence on the outcome variable. In short, if you have reason to think that uncontrolled variables (either from the setting or from the way the study was set up) were allowed to influence the outcome variable, you should also question the portrayal of treatment effectiveness depicted by the study's findings.

Statistical Conclusion Validity. Statistical conclusion validity, which is another aspect of credibility, has to do with the proper use of statistical analysis in reaching conclusions about the data (Cook and Campbell, 1979). The most common threats to statistical conclusion validity are low statistical power, use of measures with low reliability, and statistical "fishing." If the sample size of a study was not large enough, a statistical result may indicate "no association between variables" or "no difference between groups." In reality, there may be an association or difference, but the study design was not powerful enough to detect it. Thus, an inadequate sample size can lead to low statistical power, which in turn produces an *erroneous* statistical conclusion. This type of conclusion error is called Type II error and is addressed in most basic research books. The use of instruments with low reliability can also lead the researcher to falsely conclude that no association or difference exists; they do so by producing a great deal of random variation in the measurements, which decreases the ability of the statistical test to detect an association or difference that really is there.

Another threat to statistical conclusion validity is likely when multiple statistical tests are conducted on the data (for example, when there are multiple dependent variables or when multiple correlation coefficients are calculated); these situations produce a high likelihood that one of the tests will be statistically significant just by chance. Cook and Campbell (1979) called this statistical fishing and recognized it as a common cause of Type I error, that is, concluding that there is an association or difference when in reality the finding is a chance occurrence. There are statistical techniques for adjusting the analysis when multiple tests are being calculated, and researchers should use them to avoid findings that have low statistical conclusion validity.

In qualitative studies, thematic conclusion validity is of concern. Thematic conclusion validity is the confidence we have that the themes or patterns that the researcher created from the data faithfully reflect what the participants said and meant, or what actually occurred, and are not the result of the researcher's preconceptions. Although it is true that all themes and patterns are interpretations, some more clearly are derived from the data than others. The researcher establishes this derivation by providing readers of the report with a clear description of how she logically moved from quotations and observations to slightly more abstract categories and then to more abstract patterns, and themes. In addition, the researcher supports her derivation by providing examples of this data transformation to show that the themes are rooted in the data, thus they are indeed valid representations of actual statements, dialogue, events, and processes.

External Validity. External validity refers to the extent to which the findings of the study can be generalized to patients, providers, settings, and time beyond those represented in the study. The findings of a study will have low external validity if (a) the sample was extremely homogeneous, (b) the sample was composed of volunteers, (c) the setting in which the research was done might have made the participants particularly responsive to one of the treatments being evaluated, or (d) the way in which the intervention was delivered was so intricate that it could not be carried out in most clinical situations. Questions related to the generalizability of findings to your specific situation have been incorporated into the appraisal of findings under the applicability profile.

An example of limited generalizability caused by the choice of sample would be a study in which only elderly people who came to an urban, senior citizen center were interviewed about their perceptions of health. The findings of such a study would have low external validity because the sample is not likely to be representative of any larger population of older persons, either by age, ethnicity, life-style, functional capabilities, geographic location, socioeconomic status, or personal characteristics. In contrast, if the sample of the study were randomly selected from seniors in a variety of living situations (living alone, with spouse or partner, in shelters, in an assisted living residence, and in a nursing home) in several areas of a city, the findings about perceptions of health could then be broadly generalized to city dwelling seniors. Moreover, if the sample were selected from city, suburban, small town, and rural communities across the country and included persons in a variety of living situations, the findings could be generalized to seniors in the United States even more broadly. Some studies are designed to have narrow generalizability, whereas others are designed for broad generalizability; regardless, it should be clear to whom the findings can be generalized.

Construct Validity. Construct validity is a form of validity that has little direct applicability to appraisal of research findings; however, the term is frequently used in research reports and is important to understanding instruments that are used to measure research variables. Construct validity is a characteristic of a measurement instrument or rating tool that describes the extent to which a score, test value, or rating number faithfully portrays the state or attribute it represents. An instrument is "valid" if it faithfully and fully captures the real-world state or attribute as it was defined by the researcher. Thus, peak expiratory flow rate (PEFR), as percentage of predicted or percentage of best ever, is used in research studies to represent the degree of airway obstruction present in a person. Beyond questions pertaining to whether people will consistently produce the maximum effort required for the measurement (which is an issue of reliability of the measure) is the issue of whether PEFR is a *true* representation of airway obstruction. It could be a valid, i.e., true, measure for one purpose but not for another, or for one population but not for another. For example, it could be a valid measure of pulmonary obstruction for evaluating the severity of asthma exacerbation, but not a valid measure for adjusting medication dosage. Alternatively, it could be a valid measure in persons with asthma, but not in persons with chronic emphysema, or it could be a valid measure for adults but not for young children. Thus, the question of validity of a measure requires a definition of what is being represented as well as a specification of the conditions under which the measure is a true indicator. The issue of the validity of a measure or rating is complex, hence you undoubtedly will want to read more about it in your research text.

In summary, the word "validity" is used in combination with other words to refer to several different research notions. In this book, internal validity and statistical conclusion validity (including thematic conclusion validity) are included in credibility, external validity enters into applicability, and construct validity will be included in the appraisal of collective evidence from studies of a clinical measuring instrument (discussed in Chapter 9).

Fit with Other Sources of Evidence

A final factor that enters into the appraisal of a finding's credibility is how it fits or doesn't fit with the other sources of clinical knowledge. A surprising finding is one which you would not have predicted based on your knowledge of prior research, your clinical experience, the dominant thinking in the field, or your general knowledge of the field. The fact that a finding runs contrary to these other sources of evidence is not a reason in and of itself to judge the finding as not credible. To be credible, however, a surprise finding should have been produced by a methodologically strong study. And you would want to use extra care in appraising such a finding. It is possible, of course, that the finding you are appraising does indeed represent a breakthrough in knowledge. Thus, a combination of questioning the methodological rigor of a study and taking into consideration the congruency between the finding and prior knowledge enters into judging the credibility of a finding (Krathwohl, 1985).

Overall Judgment

The term credibility refers to the overall judgment that the conclusions the researcher reached about the relationship among the variables are likely and that other explanations of the data are unlikely. In appraising studies you will be asked whether you judge the findings to be credible. This is in a sense a "bottom line" question. To answer it you must have a deep understanding of how the study was conducted. If you answer in the positive, you mean that you think the study was reasonably well conducted and have confidence in its findings, and thus you will consider using them your practice. If you answer in the negative, you mean that you think the findings could have been a result of the way the study was designed and conducted rather than a true reflection of reality. In this case you would not have confidence in the findings and you would not want to let them shape your practice. The findings of a study can fail to earn your confidence either because the study has many minor flaws that accumulated to erode your confidence in it or because it has one serious flaw that undermined your overall confidence in its findings. The issue you must decide when appraising the credibility of a finding is: How critically flawed is the study from which the finding came?

A warning is in order here: every study has minor weaknesses and vulnerabilities—there is no such thing as a perfect study. Practitioners new to research appraisal have a tendency to be too harsh and to reject findings because the study was not ideal in all ways. You need to recognize the study's weaknesses but at the same time ask to what degree they undermine the credibility of the findings. Just as you don't want to use findings that come from a poorly designed study, you don't want to overlook findings just because the study failed to consider one or several factors of small overall consequence.

You may find yourself wanting to differentiate between "highly credible" and "moderately credible" studies. Although a case could be made for this distinction, it complicates the appraisal of evidence considerably, and it's not clear that such a distinction is possible given the nature of the review you will have the time and skill to conduct. Instead, you are asked to decide whether a study was well enough conducted to have confidence in its findings or not (yes or no), and if it was, you will proceed to consider it further.

Clinical Significance

Once you have determined that the findings of a study are credible because they were produced by reasonably sound investigative methods, you must still consider whether the results are also clinically significant, or practically meaningful. Appraising the clinical significance of results is a knotty issue, but your clinical knowledge will serve you well in this part of the appraisal. Essentially, you need to ask: Are the results sizable enough that they are clinically or practically important? For example, is the impact of a problem-solving intervention on patients' coping ability sizable enough to make a practical difference in their everyday lives? Is the mean number of *Proteus* and *E. coli* bacteria adhering to the cells of the urinary tract of persons who drank cranberry juice different enough from the mean of the control group to make a practical difference in whether persons who drink cranberry juice will experience symptoms of a urinary tract infection or not? Is the average "after score" on a 6-minute walking test different enough from the "before score" to think that a clinically meaningful functional improvement has resulted from an exercise intervention? For a group of adolescents who participated in a peer group discussion of accidents, was the reduction in the number of risky behaviors they engaged in per month enough to have a practical effect on their risk of injury or death due to an accident?

Clinical versus Statistical Significance

A study may have been well conducted and the results may have been statistically significant, yet the associations found between variables, or the advantage produced by the experimental treatment, may be too small to be of practical clinical importance. Thus, statistical significance does not automatically confer clinical significance on the results. The statistical tests used to analyze data (most commonly the t test, the F test, r coefficient, or chi-square test) and their associated significance levels (p values) indicate the likelihood that the association or difference found between variables is just a fluke—an association or difference that would not hold up with data from different samples. The closer the p value is to zero (0), the less likely the association or difference found is due to chance. This is important information for knowing how confident we can be that there really is a relationship or difference between the variables. These statistics provide an objective and recognized way of determining what level of confidence we can have in the data-based inference we are making about reality; hence, they are called inferential statistics.

However, these statistics say little about the practical size of the association between the variables or about the size of the difference between the mean of a treatment group and that of a control group. A study could find that a certain approach to increasing oral contraception adherence had a statistically significant benefit ($p = 0.03$), but upon looking at the results more carefully, you realize that even though the 40 young women who received the experimental intervention had increased their mean adherence scores from 23 out of 28 days to 25 out of 28 days, only five had achieved complete adherence (taken on time for 28 of 28 days) in two consecutive months. Even though the mean increase in compliance days was more than that achieved by the group who received standard care, you still have to ask whether this difference is sufficient to produce dependable protection against conception.

In contrast, some results may not be statistically significant yet may be clinically significant. In a study examining the effects of a home-based arm exercise training intervention for persons with chronic lung diseases, the authors concluded that statistically a difference in the ability to perform arm work was not documented (Bauldoff, Hoffman, Sciurba, and Zullo, 1996). Yet, when one considers the average arm endurance score before and at two times after the training intervention, and particularly when one compares

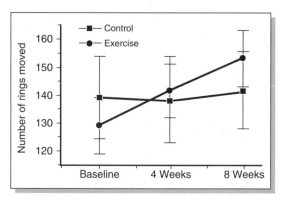

Figure 7–1. Number of rings moved by exercise and control groups during Celli upper-extremity endurance test. Graph shows baseline values and measurements at 4 and 8 weeks. (From Bauldoff, G.S., Hoffmann, L.A., Sciurba, F., and Zullo, T.G. (1996). Home-based, upper-arm exercise training for patients with chronic obstructive pulmonary disease. *Heart and Lung, 25*:291.)

the training group's scores to the control group's, it is clear that the exercise group improved considerably, whereas the control group remained essentially unchanged (Fig. 7–1). The benefit did not reach statistical significance because the sample size was so small ($n = 20$), but the results clearly show that the intervention is very promising and is deserving of study using a larger sample in which the effect of the intervention would have a better chance of being demonstrated. Even though the results were not statistically significant at the $p = 0.05$ level, from a clinical perspective the data indicate that there is good reason to believe that the intervention can improve the exercise endurance of persons with chronic lung disease.

Ultimately, the appraisal decision regarding clinical significance is a personal judgment. The appraiser should have a solid rationale for the judgment, and the rationale should rest on experience with the clinical situation, on a recognized maxim, on research-based knowledge from another study, or on patients' values.

Making Clinical Sense of the Results

You should not rely solely on the statistical tests and probability levels to make sense of the data; instead, you should also try to make clinical sense of the data. Oddly, data in research reports are often not reported in ways that answer the questions practitioners have. However, by examining the tables that display grouped data in the report you may be able to find answers to your questions. Even though the researcher didn't do it in the report, you may find it beneficial to create a visual display of the data that will be useful to you, e.g., a 2×2 table like the one shown in Table 7–2 or

| | | Completely Adherent for 2 Consecutive | Number of |
Intervention Group	Nonadherent	Months	Participants
Experimental approach	35 (87.5%)	5 (12.5%)	40
Standard approach	38 (95%)	2 (5%)	40

Table 7–2. **Hypothetical Study Results**

a line graph displaying scores at various points in time (with scores on the vertical axis and time on the horizontal axis) as shown in Figure 7–1.

Another way to make clinical sense of the data is to focus on the measures of clinical significance (also called measures of clinical efficacy) reported in the study, rather than on the statistics. The most commonly reported measures of clinical significance are: absolute risk reduction, numbers needed to treat, relative risk, and relative risk reduction. These measures will be explained in detail in a subsequent section of this chapter, but if you are not already familiar with them, for now you just need to know that they are arithmetic ways of presenting the data that convey the size of the benefit that can be expected from a particular way of doing something when compared to another way of doing it. Consider a study of parents of newborns who had access via phone or via e-mail to a resource person at set times every day. The measures of clinical significance portrayed would indicate whether off-hours trips to an emergency department and calls to a pediatrician or pediatric nurse practitioner could be reduced from 10 percent over a 2-month period for usual care parents to a target level of less than 5 percent for special access parents. In addition, these ways of portraying the data could indicate the number of persons who would need to be provided with this special access in order to eliminate one off-hours contact. Clearly, data presented in this way would be useful to pediatric care practices considering implementing a call-in time and e-mail access for new parents, as it would indicate in very practical, real-world terms how much benefit could be expected with the new service. If researchers do not report data using these measures of clinical significance, it may be possible for you to calculate these measures yourself (as described later in this chapter).

In short, you may need to set the statistics aside for a minute and consider the clinical meaning of the results so as to link the results to their real-world implications; this will require you to think about the data from a logical, clinical perspective, rather than a statistical perspective. The questions in the clinical significance subsets will assist you in assuming this perspective.

Applicability

Even when you decide that a study's findings are credible and clinically significant, you still must ask, "Should I attempt to incorporate them into my practice?" Thoughtful consideration of whether and how to apply research findings has a long history in the nursing literature on research-based practice. In 1979, Haller, Reynolds, and Horsely wrote, "Even under ideal conditions of clinical control, utilization of research in the clinical setting constitutes a change in the independent variable" (p. 50). Thus, the question of applicability of findings takes appraisal beyond consideration of the methods by which the findings were produced and beyond consideration of the clinical meaning of the findings to consideration of whether the findings, e.g., desirable patient outcomes, are likely to be realized in a particular clinical setting.

Rationale for Changing or Not Changing

The reasons for making a change based on the findings of a single study include the following: the findings were derived from a sample of patients similar to those you see, the action found effective by the study would be safe and feasible to implement, and the treatment effect was quite large and as a result is likely to hold up under conditions of everyday practice. There are also many good reasons for not making a change. One such reason would be that the sample on which the findings were obtained was quite different from the people for whom you provide care, hence you have reason to believe that the findings may not hold up with your patients. Similarly, if a subgroup of those studied that is similar to the patients you see did not respond as well to the therapy as the group on average did, you would most likely decide not to adopt the therapy. Another reason would be that you or your agency think that you would not be able to use the finding in a way that will achieve the same effects or outcomes given your resources, the skill level of your staff, or the values and socioeconomic resources of your patient population.

If adopting a research-based intervention or therapy would involve some degree of risk to the patient, you may decide that you would rather wait for another study to evaluate the benefit-risk trade-off or to get a more precise estimate of the magnitude of the treatment effect. Similarly, if implementing the study's findings would involve abandoning a therapy which you believe works well or would involve a considerable investment of resources, you may decide to not make a change at this time. As these mediating factors indicate, there are many good reasons for deciding not to change one's practice based on a particular study; you should not feel compelled to immediately change your practice because a sound study demonstrated the effectiveness of an intervention in a particular sample under a certain set of circumstances.

In brief, the research may provide sound support for the efficacy of a certain intervention, but you must decide if the intervention is likely to be feasible, safe, and effective in your situation. The concern in transferring research findings into clinical practice is that the transference may involve changes, or differences in conditions, that extend beyond the limits of what the research actually tested, and thus the findings may not hold up under the new conditions.

Nature of the Change

To help you think specifically about what changes you are considering, you will be asked to consider whether the change in practice you are making is substantial, incremental, or soft. Substantial changes typically involve acquiring new skills, purchasing new equipment, or revising the way care is provided, e.g., a new protocol or clinical pathway. Incremental change involves changing a particular action or adding an element to your approach rather than adopting a whole new approach. A study of physician behavior change in which 775 changes described by 340 physicians were analyzed revealed that 62 percent of the changes made were incremental in nature (Fox, Mazmanian, and Putnam, 1989). An example of an incremental change would be the decision to apply pressure to the site for 10 seconds prior to giving an intramuscular injection (Barnhill, Holbert, Jackson, and Erickson, 1996). This change is incremental because only one action would be added to the procedure rather than changing the entire way in which intramuscular injections are given.

"Soft" usage occurs when a reader takes enough note of a research finding to let it influence his understanding or thinking about a certain kind of situation, or when the information is just "stored" for future use without a specific plan to change practice. Among clinical nurse specialists, soft usage was the most frequent type of research utilization (Stetler and DiMaggio, 1991). An example of a soft change is the practitioner who reads a study about chest pain among African-American women (Fisher, Cooper, Weber, and Liao, 1997) and acquires knowledge and insights about the psychosocial factors associated with the occurrence of both cardiac and noncardiac chest pain. Even though the findings of this study do not directly address how to differentiate between the two types of pain, they do identify issues that should be explored when evaluating chest pain in African-American women. The practitioner who reads this study will be more sensitive to verbal clues and information suggestive of stress in these women's lives, and may change just slightly how she asks questions when interviewing them. Even though the research did not validate a whole new assessment approach or discrete intervention, it does have the potential to change how care is enacted, thereby making it research-based to a greater extent than it was before the practitioner read the study. Awareness of the kind of change you are making may help keep your effort in perspective as well as recognize the "little ways" in which you are influenced by research.

Planning and Evaluating the Change

If you decide to make a change in your practice, the last few questions of the application profile ask you to think through how you will go about making the change, and once the change has been made, how you will know if patients have benefited. A clinical evaluation plan does not mean you will have to conduct research, but it does mean you will need to think about how you can practically and systematically evaluate if your patients are responding well to the new intervention or change in practice. Ideas for how you might evaluate their responses are presented in Chapter 11; you may want to briefly look at those before proceeding to the next chapter.

In summary, the activities that must be performed in appraising the findings of an original study involve (a) getting a sense of what was studied, how it was studied, and what was found; (b) forming a judgment regarding the credibility of the findings; (c) deciding whether the results are clinically significant; and (d) deciding whether and how the findings could be applied in your practice. These activities form the basis of the four subsets of questions that compose each set of appraisal questions.

MEASURES OF CLINICAL SIGNIFICANCE: FURTHER EXPLANATION

There are several reasons for devoting special attention to the measures by which the clinical significance of results can be appraised. First, the journals of health care disciplines other than medicine are not using these measures of clinical significance extensively in their reporting of research; thus, definition and explanation of them are needed to familiarize practitioners with them. (In the field of medicine the terms "measures of clinical efficacy" or "treatment effect" are used to refer to measures that compare the size of the effect of an experimental method of treatment to that of a control group or standard treatment). Second, because many journals are not reporting research using the measures of clinical significance, readers may have to calculate these measures by themselves.

Even though you may not be familiar with the measures of clinical significance, you will undoubtedly not find them difficult to understand because they involve ways of thinking that are very much like those you use in everyday practice when deciding that a treatment approach is working or not working with a patient, or with one of the subpopulations in your practice. Measures of clinical significance are arithmetic ways of presenting results so that they have clinical meaning. The measures used in the medical literature to convey a practical sense of how a treatment compares to a control or standard treatment are: absolute risk reduction, numbers needed to treat, relative risk reduction, and relative risk. Two other useful measures are the difference in the mean scores of the groups being compared and the coefficient of determination when dealing with correlational results.

Dichotomous Data

It is easier to appraise the clinical significance of results when an intervention (such as method of rewarming patients after surgery) or a risk factor (such as level of exercise) is being evaluated, and when the outcome variable is reported in dichotomous terms. Dichotomous means that an outcome is characterized by one of two states or outcome categories. In reality, we often think of health outcomes in dichotomous terms: patients improve or don't improve with a certain therapy, they return to work or don't return to work, they live or they die, they gain the ability to walk 50 feet without assistance or they don't, they increase their self-care knowledge by a meaningful amount or they don't, they follow recommended regimens or they don't, they experience a complication/side effect or they don't.

Our frequent use of dichotomous data has its origins in the limited amount of memory space available to most mortal humans. It is just easier to remember whether an event occurred or didn't, or whether a clinical value was above or below a meaningful cut-off point than to remember the exact numerical value. For example, persons may qualify for assisted living based on whether their activities of daily living score is above a certain point, or a person who has had a renal transplant may be considered at risk for organ rejection because his score on an assessment tool for organ rejection risk after transplant is above a previously set point score. We find it easier to remember whether or not a person qualified for admission to assisted living than to remember his activities of daily living score. Some clinical categories are based on assessment tool cut-off points that have been established somewhat arbitrarily, but increasingly, cut-off points for being considered "at risk" are based on research. Working with clinical categories rather than values on some unit of measurement, although not always adequate, may save memory space and make clinical communication easier because categories are often easier to interpret and easier to remember than a data value. In addition, they go beyond numbers to assign clinical meaning to the data.

Other Views of the Data

Even though the dependent variable in a study is continuous in nature, the researcher may provide frequency data regarding how many people with each treatment achieved and didn't achieve a certain clinically meaningful level of the outcome. When this is provided, a reader can easily calculate one of the measures of clinical significance. Consider again the hypothetical study mentioned earlier in this chapter about an experimental intervention designed to improve young women's adherence to taking daily oral contraceptives (see Table 7–2). The mean improvement in days of adherence was statistically significant, indicating that the experimental intervention was more effective than the standard approach. However, the researcher could also provide other perspectives on the data which would be clinically more meaningful.

The following four statements provide a sense of the kind of information conveyed about the data by the measures of clinical significance. The calculations of these measures are explained in the next section.

1. The difference (in percentage) between the standard intervention group's rate of nonadherence and the experimental group's rate is 7.5 percent; thus, absolute risk reduction (ARR) of nonadherence = 7.5 percent.
2. Thirteen (13) persons would need to be treated with the experimental treatment rather than the standard treatment to prevent one person from becoming nonadherent; number needed to treat (NNT) = 13.
3. Persons receiving the experimental intervention were 92 percent as likely to be nonadherent as those receiving the standard treatment; relative risk (RR) of nonadherence = 92 percent.
4. Relative to the standard treatment, the experimental treatment reduced nonadherence by 8 percent; relative risk reduction (RRR) of nonadherence = 8 percent.

Clearly these measures of clinical effect provide perspectives on the effect of the treatment that are not provided by the hypothesis testing statement "The experimental intervention had a statistically significant benefit on nonadherence," or even by the table. These measures provide you with practical information about *how much* the intervention affected nonadherence.

Definitions and Calculations

The size of the treatment's effect can be portrayed using any one of the measures of clinical significance,[1] all of which are easy to calculate.

1. The absolute risk reduction (ARR) is the difference in proportions between those who experienced an adverse outcome (in this case, nonadherence) with the standard care versus the percentage of those who did with experimental care (ARR = .95 − .875 = 0.075 = 7.5 percent).

---

[1]The measures of clinical significance described in this book are point estimates based on the data in the study; many investigators who report these measures report them as point estimates with the 95 percent confidence intervals around them. This is the most informative way of reporting as it provides the range within which the true effect is likely to lie (Guyatt, Sackett, and Cook, 1994).

2. The number needed to treat (NNT) is the number of patients that need to be treated using the experimental treatment to prevent one bad outcome (NNT = 1/ARR = 1/0.075 = 13.3). NNT is particularly useful because it incorporates both baseline improvement with standard treatment and the increase realized with the experimental treatment, thereby telling the practitioner in concrete terms "how much effort they must expend to prevent [or achieve] one event" (Laupacis, Sackett, and Roberts, 1988, p. 1730).

3. The relative risk or risk ratio (RR) is the ratio of those who experienced a bad outcome with the experimental intervention to those who experienced the bad outcome with standard care (a ratio of 1 would mean that the treatments are equal in preventing the bad outcome) (RR = 0.875/0.95 = 0.92); this means that persons receiving the experimental treatment were 92 percent as likely to be a nonadherent case as those receiving the standard treatment.

4. Relative risk reduction (RRR) is the proportion of risk reduction associated with the experimental treatment relative to that occurring in the standard care group: RRR = (0.95 − 0.875)/0.95 = 0.08.[2] Thus, the experimental treatment produced an 8 percent relative reduction in nonadherence.

These measures of clinical significance are based on avoidance of the adverse outcome of nonadherence, but could just as easily be cast in the positive as bringing about the positive outcome of adherence. In brief, if the data consisted of dichotomous outcomes or if the results were converted to dichotomous outcomes and frequencies in the report, these measures of clinical significance can be used to determine the magnitude of effect the intervention had on a clinical outcome of interest—hence, they help make clinical sense of the results. For another example of how to calculate these measures and further discussion of them, see Appendix C.

Difference in Group Means

If the data in a treatment-outcome study is not presented in dichotomous terms, you can appraise its clinical significance by examining the difference between the means of the groups compared and considering its implications from a clinical perspective. Many reports include a table that displays the means and standard deviations for each treatment group on each dependent variable; such a table provides all the information you need to consider the difference in outcomes from a clinical perspective.

---

[2]RRR may also be calculated as 1 − RR; in the example the RRR would be calculated as 1 − 0.92 = 0.08 = 8 percent.

Examples of Difference in Means

In a hypothetical study aimed at evaluating the effect of an instructional intervention designed to increase parents' use of analgesia with children at home after outpatient surgery, the control group received an average of 2.2 doses of analgesia per day for the first three days after surgery, whereas the experimental group received an average of 3.1 doses. Would you consider that increase a clinically meaningful difference in response to the intervention? The difference in means resulting from the intervention in comparison to the control groups may at first seem small, but upon more thought, you will realize that even one more dose of analgesic in a 24-hour period could reduce a child's discomfort considerably. This example illustrates that a simple way to appraise the clinical significance of results is to think about the benefit achieved from a clinical perspective by asking, "Is this amount of difference (benefit) likely to have any meaningful effect on the patient's well-being or clinical outcomes?"

Another example is a study in which patients were randomly assigned to three different ways of rewarming during postanesthesia recovery (Guiffre, Finnie, Lynam, and Smith, 1991); see Table 7–3 as reprinted from that report. The mean difference in number of minutes to achieve a temperature of 36°C between the use of warm blankets and the use of forced warm air was 41 minutes (153.1 minus 112.2 minutes). In other words, on average, the patients warmed with forced warm air achieved 36°C 41 minutes faster than did the patients in the group warmed with blankets. From a clinical perspective this could be an important difference in that it would allow patients to meet criteria for discharge from the recovery area and return to their rooms earlier, saving the discomforts of being in the recovery area as well as some of the high financial cost of being there. It must be recognized, however, that this mean difference is a point estimate of how much faster patients warm with forced warm air rather than warm blankets.

Table 7–3. **Mean Number of Minutes (SD) It Took Patients in the Three Groups to Warm to 36°C (96.8°F) and to Meet Discharge Criteria**

	Minutes to 36°C (96.8°F)		Minutes to Discharge Criteria Met	
	N	Min (SD)	N	Min (SD)
Blankets	31	153.1 (77.8)	30	238.8 (97.2)
Lights	30	148.7 (81.6)	30	240.5 (133.4)
Warm air	29	112.2 (52.3)	28	217.9 (109.9)
P	0.06		0.71	

Source: Data taken from Guiffre, M., Finnie, J., Lynam, D.A., and Smith, D. (1991). *Journal of Post Anesthesia Nursing, 6*:392, Table 2.

The Value of Confidence Intervals

Using the point estimate of difference in means of the two groups being compared, may or may not be an accurate indication of what the magnitude of difference might be if the entire population participated in the study[3]; in a study with a small sample size the point estimate is likely to *not* be precise. A better approach is to rely on a confidence interval around the point estimate of the difference in the means. Confidence intervals around a mean difference, and around the other measures of clinical significance, are very helpful in determining how precise the point estimate is. They provide another angle on the data that helps in deciding whether the results are clinically significant. If the 95 percent confidence interval is narrow, the point estimate is a precise indicator of likely benefit. However, if a confidence interval is quite wide, the true value of the measure of clinical effect, be it mean difference, relative risk, or any of the other measures of clinical significance, may not be close to the point estimate.

Continuing with the rewarming example just presented, the 95 percent confidence interval around the difference in the means between the two ways of rewarming was calculated to be 6.44 minutes to 75.36 minutes to achieve a temperature of 36°C.[4] This is quite a wide difference and indicates a high degree of imprecision in the point estimate of 41 minutes' difference in rewarming time with the two methods. (This wide confidence interval is undoubtedly due to the relatively large variability of scores within groups.) The confidence interval conveys the information that rewarming with forced warm air may really take anywhere between 6 minutes and 75 minutes less. Clearly a 6-minute gain in rewarming time would not be clinically important but a 75-minute gain would be quite important. The fact that the 95 percent confidence interval is so wide makes it almost impossible to estimate the amount of time benefit that would actually be realized by using the forced warm air method rather than warm blankets. Had a larger sample been used, the confidence interval around the mean difference in rewarming time undoubtedly would have been narrower; hence the practitioner considering implementation of the forced warm air method would have had a more precise estimate of how much faster patients in his population who are rewarmed this way would achieve 36°C. Nevertheless, the consideration of the mean difference and particularly the 95 percent confidence interval

---

[3]Although the point estimate is the single best estimate of the unknown population value, it is still an educated guess based on the data from a single sample (Gardner and Altman, 1986; Huck and Cormier, 1996).

[4]The confidence interval around the difference in the means is not provided in the report, but it was calculated from the data in the report. The statistical result of the report is slightly different from that of the confidence interval (the omnibus F was not significant at the $p = 0.05$ level whereas the 95 percent confidence interval does not include zero). Such contradictory results are due to sampling error (Nichols, 1998).

around that mean difference point estimate provides important information for deciding whether a finding is clinically important or not.

It is prudent to calculate confidence intervals around any difference in means that you are considering,[5] rather than relying on a point estimate of the difference; however, calculations will often be required. Although the calculations are not that difficult, you may elect not to calculate a 95 percent confidence interval, and to just rely on the point estimate of the difference in the means. Should you choose not to calculate a 95 percent confidence interval around the difference in the mean, you should at least keep the following general rule in mind: If the study had a small sample size or used instruments with low reliability, the confidence interval around the difference between means is likely to be imprecise, i.e., wide, and should be viewed as only a very rough indicator of what the true difference in mean would be if the entire population were used in the study.

The formula for constructing a 95 percent confidence interval around a difference in means and the calculations that went into determining it for the rewarming example are provided in Appendix D. Once you spend a little time with this formula and example, you will realize that it is not that difficult to calculate a confidence interval around a mean difference based on point estimates. And once mastered, this will be a powerful tool for appraising the clinical significance of findings where means of groups are reported.

Coefficient of Determination

The last measure of clinical significance that will be discussed is the coefficient of determination (r^2). Although not as direct a measure of clinical significance as those previously presented, r^2 does provide a practical perspective on the covariation between two variables when the covariation is reported as Pearson Correlation Coefficients (r). The value of r^2, which is calculated by squaring r, indicates the proportion of variability in y scores that is associated with the x scores as well as the proportion of variability in x scores that is associated with the y scores (the two proportions are identical). The value of r^2 will always fall between 0 and 1.00, with an r^2 value of 1.00 indicating that all of the variability in each variable is attributable to the other variable, and the value close to zero indicating very little association between the two variables. An example would be a study in which the association between weight and height is of interest but neither is considered causal of the other. Clearly, weight and height are strongly associated but they are not perfectly correlated. If the r value indicating the relationship between them in a sample of persons were 0.76, then the r^2 value depicting

---

[5]Other formulas are used to calculate confidence intervals around single means, proportions, and their differences (Altman, 1997).

their relationship in that group would be 0.58 (0.76 squared). This value of r^2 means that 58 percent of the variability in height is associated with weight while 58 percent of the variability in weight is associated with height; it also means that 42 percent of the variability in both height and weight is associated with other variables (100 percent minus 58 percent equals 42 percent). Thus, squaring a Pearson Correlation Coefficient *(r)* provides a practical perspective on the meaning of *r* because it indicates how strongly the two variables influence one another as well as the extent to which other variables influence them.

In more complex correlational studies when there is a directional hypothesis proposing one or several independent variables that influence a dependent variable, coefficients of determination are also reported. In simple regression analysis (when there is one independent variable and one dependent variable), the r^2 value indicates the proportion of the dependent variable that is attributable to the independent variable. Similarly, in multiple regression analysis (when there are two or more independent variables and one dependent variable), the R^2 value indicates the proportion of the dependent variable that is attributable to the independent variables. For example, the independent variables of height, gender, and average daily caloric intake taken together might predict 74 percent of the variability in weight (the dependent variable) in a particular group of people ($R^2 = 0.74$).

Small values for r^2 and R^2 should not be dismissed out-of-hand, however, as they may be clinically significant when their effect on patient outcomes is considered. In addition, when considered at the population level, a small amount of explained variance can potentially translate to an important difference in outcomes (Rosnow and Rosenthal, 1993). In descriptive correlational studies, coefficients of determination (r^2) may or may not be reported but can be easily calculated by squaring Pearson Correlation Coefficients *(r)*. In predictive studies in which the data were analyzed using simple or multiple regression analysis, the r^2 or the R^2 for a specified set of predictor variables is almost always reported. In summary, r^2 and R^2 have a more clear practical meaning than do some of the other statistics used to analyze the relationships that exist between and among variables.

SUMMARY

Appraisal questions for each of the five types of study designs are grouped into synopsis, credibility profile, clinical significance profile, and application profile subsets. The synopsis subset questions require you to recognize the elements of the study and to get a sense of what was studied, how the study was conducted, and what the findings were. The credibility profile questions will help you challenge the credibility of the study's findings, that is, to evaluate their internal validity and statistical conclusion validity. You will be required to make an overall judgment decision regarding the credibility of the findings. The clinical significance questions will help you decide if the associations found in the data are of enough magnitude to be considered clinically important or not; a focus on, or calculation of, at least one measure of clinical significance is advocated. The applicability profile subset of questions pertains to whether you should change your current way of doing things. They require you to consider the applicability of the findings to your specific situation as well as the feasibility of adopting the methods or knowledge confirmed by the research.

Unfortunately, not all research reports provide a measure of clinical significance, but increasingly, studies are reporting results using them and confidence intervals around them. Therefore, it behooves all practitioners to become comfortable with the measures of clinical significance because understanding of them is critical to determining the clinical significance of research results (Guyatt, Sackett, Cook and the Evidence-Based Medicine Working Group, 1994; Sackett, Richardson, Rosenberg, and Haynes, 1997). The same is true for the use of confidence intervals—if you aren't comfortable with their interpretation and why they provide better information than point estimates alone, you will want to refer to a statistics book or a clinical article about interpreting them (Gardner and Altman, 1986; Glantz, 1997; Huck and Cormier, 1996; Munro, 1997).

The decision to use a research finding must consider all aspects of the finding—its credibility, its clinical significance, and its applicability to your patient or setting. It is a decision involving judgment at several points. Surely, you want to make it objectively and logically, but even with the sets of questions provided, the decision will not always be clear. Two practitioners using the questions to appraise a finding (or findings) may arrive at different conclusions regarding the credibility of the finding or about whether, or how, to change practice, just as two trained and certified appraisers of antiques may arrive at quite different conclusions regarding an item's worth. Ultimately, of course, practice should rarely be changed on the basis of one study. Instead, the practitioner should appraise findings across several studies, which is similar to getting several estimates of an antique's value before deciding on a fair price.

References

Altman, D.G. (1997). Appendix: Confidence intervals. *In* D.L. Sackett, W.S. Richardson, W. Rosenberg, and R.B. Haynes, *Evidence-based Medicine: How to Practice and Teach EBM* (pp. 227–234). New York: Churchill Livingstone.

Badger, T.A. (1993). Physical health impairment and depression among older adults. *IMAGE: Journal of Nursing Scholarship, 25*:325–330.

Barnhill, B.J., Holbert, M.D., Jackson, N.M., and Erickson, R.S. (1996). Using pressure to decrease the pain of intramuscular injections. *Journal of Pain and Symptom Management, 12*:52–58.

Bauldoff, G.S., Hoffman, L.A., Sciurba, F., and Zullo, T.G. (1996). Home-based, upper-arm exercise training for patients with chronic obstructive pulmonary disease. *Heart and Lung, 25*:288–294.

Brown, S.A., and Grimes, D.E. (1993). *Nurse Practitioners and Certified Nurse-Midwives: A Meta-Analysis of Studies on Nurses in Primary Care Roles.* Washington, DC: American Nurses Publishing.

Cook, T.D., and Campbell, D.T. (1979). *Quasi-Experimentation: Design and Analysis Issues for Field Studies.* Boston: Houghton Mifflin.

Cooper, H.M. (1982). Scientific guidelines for conducting integrative research reviews. *Review of Educational Research, 52*:291–302.

Fisher, S.G., Cooper, R., Weber, L., and Liao, Y. (1997). Psychosocial correlates of chest pain among African-American women. *Women and Health, 24*:19–35.

Gardner, M.J., and Altman, D.G. (1986). Confidence intervals rather than P values: Estimation rather than hypothesis testing. *British Medical Journal, 292*:746–750.

Glantz, S.A. (1997). *Primer of Biostatistics, 4th ed.* New York: McGraw-Hill.

Guiffre, M., Finnie, J., Lynam, D.A., and Smith, D. (1991). Rewarming postoperative patients: Lights, blankets, or forced warm air. *Journal of Post Anesthesia Nursing, 6*:387–393.

Guyatt, G.H., Sackett, D.L., Cook, D.J., and the Evidence-Based Medicine Work Group (1994). Users' guides to the medical literature; How to use an article about therapy or prevention, What were the results and will they help me in caring for my patients? *Journal of the American Medical Association, 271*:59–63

Heller, K.B., Reynolds, M.A., and Horsley, J.A. (1979). Developing research-based innovation protocols. *Research in Nursing and Health, 2,* 45–51

Huck, S.W., and Cormier, W.H. (1986). *Reading Statistics and Research, 2nd ed.* New York: HarperCollins.

Kearney, M.H., Murphy, S., Irwin, K., and Rosenbaum, M. (1995). Salvaging self: A grounded theory of pregnancy on crack cocaine. *Nursing Research, 44*:208–213.

Krathwohl, D.R. (1985). Social and behavioral science research: A new framework for conceptualizing, implementing, and evaluating research studies. San Francisco: Jossey-Bass.

Meydani, S.N., Meydani, M., Blumberg, J.B., Leka, L.S., Siber, G., Loszewski, R., Thompson, C., Pedrosa, M.C., Diamond, R.D., and Stollar, D. (1997). Vitamin E supplementation and in vivo immune response in healthy elderly subjects. *Journal of American Medical Association, 277*:1380–1386.

Munro, B.H. (1997). *Statistical Methods for Health Care Research, 3rd ed.* Philadelphia: Lippincott.

Nichols, D.P. (1998). My tests don't agree. *SPSS Keywords, 66,* 5.

Pickler, R.H., Higgins, K.E., and Crummette, B.D. (1993). The effect of nonnutritive sucking on bottle-feeding stress in preterm infants. *Journal of Gynecology and Neonatal Nursing, 22*:230–234.

Rosnow, R.L., and Rosenthal, R. (1993). *Beginning Behavioral Research: A Conceptual Primer.* New York: Macmillan.

Stetler, C.B. (1994). Refinement of the Stetler/Marram model for application of research findings to practice. *Nursing Outlook, 42*:15–25.

Stetler, C.B., and DiMaggio, G. (1991). Research utilization among clinical nurse specialists. *Clinical Nurse Specialist, 5*:151–155.

Valdini, A., and Cargill, L.C. (1997). Access and barriers to mammography in New England community health centers. *The Journal of Family Practice, 15*:243–249.

Appraising Findings from Single Original Studies

Appraisal of a single original study is one of the pathway options that can be taken when seeking research evidence on which to base practice (see Figure 8–1). Appraisal of several, or even many, original studies is an early step on the collective evidence pathway, i.e., when two or more studies are available. In this chapter appraisal questions are provided for five types of studies: qualitative research studies, descriptive studies, studies using correlational designs, those using randomized experimental designs, and studies using quasi-experimental designs. The chapter is divided into sections for each type of design; in each section issues relevant to the particular design are addressed and a set of appraisal questions is provided. The questions incorporate the standards by which each type of study should be considered scientifically credible and issues that determine whether or not to make a change in practice based on the findings. Rather than read straight through this chapter, you may prefer to read the section that applies to a study you want to appraise. Later, when you have a study of a different type, you can read the appropriate section for that study. You may also want to refer to your research text for a different perspective on the issues involved in appraising the scientific soundness of studies using a particular research method.

LOGISTICS

To select the most appropriate set of appraisal questions, you first must determine the research design that was used for the study under consider-

Pathways of Research-based Practice

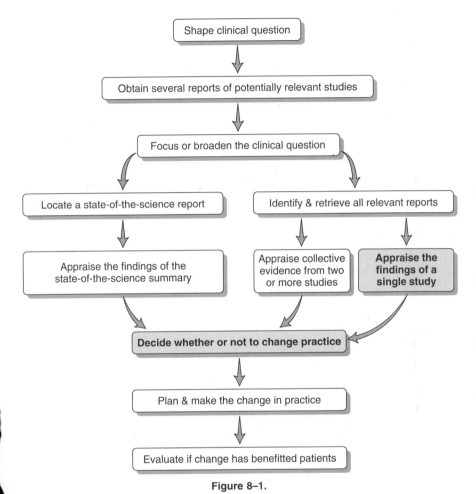

Figure 8–1.

ation. A decision algorithm is provided in Figure 8–2[1] to assist you in making this selection; following the algorithm from the top will lead you to a decision about the design used. To answer the questions in the algorithm you will first need to familiarize yourself with the study's research questions and with its design features. Sometimes reading the abstract will provide this information, whereas other times you will have to extract the design features from the Methods section. Some researchers will name the design used at

---

[1]This algorithm serves the specific purpose of deciding which of the five sets of appraisal questions provided in this chapter to use; it should not be considered as a definitive categorization of research designs.

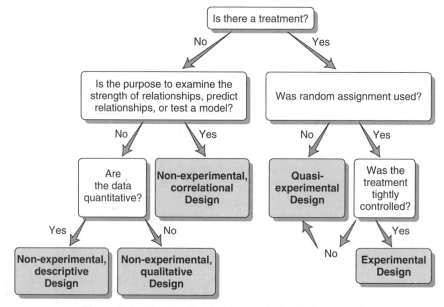

Figure 8–2. Algorithm for deciding on design that was used.

the beginning of the Methods section or in the statement of the study's purpose, which may make the use of the algorithm unnecessary. Unfortunately, the labels used to refer to research designs vary greatly; thus, the label the author used may not be in agreement with your view of the design that was actually used or with the definitions of design types used in this book. You must also realize that some studies do not fit clearly and completely into one design category; rather, they have features of several design types. When appraising studies with mixed designs, you will have to decide which set of appraisal questions will work best or consider using two sets of appraisal questions.

If only one study on a question of interest is available, you will have to decide whether or not to change your practice based on that one study. In that case you should complete all four subsets of questions: synopsis, credibility profile, clinical significance profile, and applicability profile. More often, however, several relevant studies will be available, requiring you to appraise the collective evidence from several or many studies. Appraisal of collective evidence begins with the appraisal of the findings of each single study, and proceeds to appraisal of the findings as a group. Hence, if you will be doing a collective appraisal, you need only complete the first three subsets of questions for a single, original study, as the application subset will be placed by a set of questions for application of collective evidence. Instead answering the application subset of questions, fill in one row of the Collective Findings Table (included in Appendix I) at this time; this will considerably

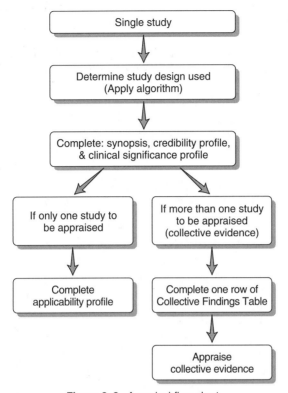

Figure 8–3. Appraisal flow chart.

facilitate the collective evidence appraisal, particularly if you will be appraising a large number of studies. Figure 8–3 illustrates how these logistics are slightly different depending on whether you will be appraising one study or more than one.

The appraisal questions were designed to help you think analytically and critically about the study, but do not lead you directly to an appraisal conclusion as critique guidelines using point systems do. The appraisal conclusions required are judgments that are too complex to be captured using points and overall scores. Instead, the questions provided draw your attention to the features, strengths, and weaknesses of the particular type of study as well as to the clinical meaning and practical aspects of the findings. It is important that you use these questions as starting points for critically thinking about the study. Most questions were designed to require you to think about how an aspect of the study was carried out or about the meaning of a finding, but even the yes-no questions should be answered with thought about the underlying issues they raise. The three "bottom line" appraisal questions are: "Overall, are the findings credible?" "Are the findings clinically significant?" and "Should I change my practice based on these findings?" Answers to these questions should be based on deliberation about the more specific questions that led up to them.

It may be helpful at this time to examine the sample single study appraisal, collective findings table, and appraisal of collective evidence provided in Appendixes E, F, and G. The logic of these appraisals will be more evident after completing this chapter and Chapter 9, but examining them now will help you acquire a sense of where your appraisal is headed, and how the individual steps contribute to getting there.

STUDIES USING NON-EXPERIMENTAL QUALITATIVE METHODS

Understanding Qualitative Methods

When the research objective is to acquire a deep understanding of (a) patient's health-related experiences; (b) the meanings health experience and illness have for them; (c) the social processes associated with illness, or (d) characteristics of health care environments, qualitative research methods are most useful. These methods include phenomenology, ethnography, and grounded theory research (Streubert and Carpenter, 1995). The specific method used depends on the research question, but in each method the phenomenon of interest is studied as it naturally occurs and participants in the phenomenon are often interviewed in depth, and/or observed over time. In addition, the data consist of descriptions and quotations, not numerical indicators or measurements. Data are checked for accuracy, veracity, and representativeness, compared with other similar data, pondered for meaning, and eventually clustered based on similarity until patterns or themes that give meaning to the data are discovered. The themes identified are considered trustworthy if the researcher makes explicit the reasoning by which themes or patterns were derived, if the themes have been validated by participants, and if the patient sample and the contexts of the situations or data collection sites are well described (Lincoln and Guba, 1985). Sometimes, the goal of qualitative studies is to produce a detailed, insightful description, whereas other times the goal is to produce a conceptual or theoretical portrayal of the issues and processes involved in a situation or experience.

The clinical significance of findings from qualitative studies is difficult to appraise because there is no quantitative measure of clinical significance to consider. However, practitioners often respond to qualitative results by noting that they resonate, or don't resonate, with what they have experienced with patients. Alternatively, they will note that qualitative results either provide a fresh perspective in understanding a situation or that they don't add anything new. These two responses can be viewed as forms of confirmation or lack of confirmation for (a) the correspondence of the findings to the facts of experienced reality and (b) their pragmatic value. Another indicator of the clinical significance of qualitative studies is the frequency with which a certain finding occurred; in other words, what proportion of respondents referred to a certain issue? A finding that occurred in all study participants would be more clinically significant than one occurring in a small number of participants. Resonance with clinical experience and the prevalence of a finding in the sample constitute forms of support for the clinical significance of results from qualitative studies.

Appraisal Questions

Synopsis

What experience, adaptive process, social process, or environment was studied?

What was the research question?

What kinds of people or situations were studied?

How was data collected?

What procedures were used to transform the data into more general categories or themes?

What are the findings? What form did the findings take (a description, a conceptual explanation, a theory, a model)?

Credibility Profile

Were participants allowed to describe their experiences and points of view in their own words? Were extensive and carefully documented observations conducted? Were patients' diaries, transcripts of dialogue, or historical records systematically analyzed?

Were participants' quotes or vivid descriptions provided in the report?

Were sufficient cases, situations, or narrative examined to convince me that a potentially generalizable pattern was identified?

Do the researcher's conclusions flow logically from the raw data?

Did the researcher confirm the interpretations/findings with any participants?

How does this finding compare to other findings in the field?

OVERALL, IS THE FINDING CREDIBLE? Yes _____ No _____

Clinical Significance Profile

Does the finding resonate with how I have experienced the reality it is portraying?

Does this finding suggest a way of viewing a patient's situation that is significantly more sensitive, more complete, or more adequate than how I have previously thought about the situation?

Was the finding present in a majority of the cases and was it impressive as capturing an important aspect of the experience, process, or situation?

IS THE FINDING CLINICALLY SIGNIFICANT? Yes _____ No _____

Applicability Profile

How effective is my current practice? On what rationale is my current practice based?

To what groups of patients or situations can I extend this finding with confidence?

How *could* I change my practice based on this finding? Would this be a substantial, incremental, or soft change?

If I changed my practice in this way, could patients be subjected to potential harm or risk?

Are there any organizational, logistical, cost, or time barriers to changing my practice? Could they be overcome?

SHOULD I CHANGE MY PRACTICE BASED ON THIS FINDING? Yes _____ No _____

How should I go about making the change?

Once I change my practice, how will I know if patients have benefited?

STUDIES USING NON-EXPERIMENTAL DESCRIPTIVE DESIGNS

Understanding Descriptive Designs

Descriptive studies are designed to portray the characteristics of a situation or a population as they naturally occur. Some descriptive studies focus on *one variable of interest* and describe its features, prevalence, frequency, patterns of occurrence, and distribution in a population; an example of this would be a study describing gastrointestinal symptoms in middle-aged people. Other descriptive studies portray a situation or the experiences of a population by documenting *several variables of interest;* a study describing the concerns, perceived stresses, optimism, and quality of life in renal transplant patients would be an example of such a study. When a cohort (by age or a common experience) is followed over time, the study is often described as a prospective cohort study; this would be the case if the renal transplant patients were followed over a five-year period. Rather than following participants over time, researchers using a cross-sectional, descriptive design recruit participants at various stages of the experience with the intent of constructing a composite portrayal of how the experience changes over time. Thus, this design accomplishes many of the same purposes as a longitudinal design, but the study can be completed in a much shorter span of time.

In cohort studies, identifiable subgroups may exist or may emerge so that comparisons between them may be made; for example, in the study of the renal transplant cohort the concerns, perceived stresses, optimism, and quality of life of those with high expectations prior to transplantation could be compared to those with low expectations. Other comparison studies examine the differences between distinct populations such as a study in which the experiences of renal transplant patients are compared to those of liver transplant patients. When making comparisons, inferential statistics such as chi square, t-tests, and Analysis of Variance (ANOVA) are often used to determine if the differences found between groups are statistically significant or just the result of chance variation.

Survey Data

When the data are acquired through structured interviews conducted in person or via the phone or through questionnaires personally distributed or mailed to the respondents, the study is called a survey.[2] Surveys are particularly useful for collecting data about behaviors enacted in everyday life; about elements of cognitive thinking such as attitudes, opinions, intentions, reasons; about values, needs, and desires; and about demographic facts. Questionnaires, because they are anonymous, are often able to obtain reliable information about personally sensitive issues. Survey research aims to describe or explore the prevalence, distributions, and interrelations of self-reported variables in a population by sampling from the population (Aday, 1996).

If well conducted, surveys can provide a great deal of accurate and valuable information. The advantages of surveys include the breadth of information that can be obtained, their relative economy of effort and cost, and their accuracy in portraying the characteristics of a population. Disadvantages of surveys include negative reactivity of persons when asked to participate in an interview or to complete a questionnaire, the effort required to obtain an adequate response rate, the research knowledge required to develop reliable and valid interview schedules or questionnaires and to use sound sampling techniques, and the potential for superficiality if the researcher doesn't know the strategies and techniques for getting to deeper, more complex information.

Structured interviews and questionnaires inherently have many potential problems including ambiguity, misinterpretation, sequence effect, leading questions, and tendency to elicit socially desirable responses; thus, skilled construction and careful pilot testing and revision are essential. In addition, if there is a low return (or response) rate, the representativeness of the data is threatened. The concern with low return rates is that the respondents

---

[2]Technically, survey is not a research design, rather a way of collecting data for a descriptive, correlational, or quasi-experimental study (Burns and Grove, 1997).

may be quite different in important but unknown ways from the nonrespondents, and thus the responses are systematically influenced by volunteer bias.

The issue of how the group of respondents was formed is critical in appraising surveys because it determines the population to whom the findings can be generalized. First, there is the issue of how the pool of contacts was selected from the target population, and then there is the issue of how the persons who agreed to be interviewed, or who sent back questionnaires, are similar to or different from the pool of contacts. Both phases determine whether the findings represent the responses of the larger, target population. Random selection from the target population is the best way to assure that the pool of contacts is representative of the larger population; survey findings based on convenience samples should be viewed with considerable caution as it is not clear to whom the findings can be generalized.

The issue of how the actual respondents could be different from the pool of contacts is even tougher. Although there is no agreed-upon standard for a minimally acceptable response rate, 75 percent is used in some U.S. government contracts for surveys (Fowler, 1993). Response rates vary widely depending on the population being sampled and on the data collection method (phone, face-to-face interview, mail). Sometimes, demographic information about the general population may be available, making it possible to determine the extent to which the respondents resemble, at least in some ways, the population (Huck and Cormier, 1996). Often, however, survey researchers settle for surmising how the two groups might be different or similar. It is important that the researcher take into account the response rate when interpreting the results, because a low response rate is a likely source of bias.

When the size of the sample needed is statistically determined, the interview or questionnaire design is carefully planned and pilot tested, and the representativeness of the respondents is considered, the findings of survey research can provide valuable insights into how a certain group of people think or live their daily lives. Hence, it is a useful form of research for health care providers interested in exploring issues of motivation and behavior.

Appraisal Questions

Synopsis

What was the question or issue being studied?

Was there one main variable of interest or several? If one, list the features of that variable that were examined. If there were several variables of interest, list them.

Was there a clearly defined group of participants? Were subgroups of the sample compared? What two or more distinct populations were compared?

Was the sample followed over time, or was a cross-sectional design used?
If the study used survey methods, how was the sample of contacts selected?
    What percentage of the contacts responded or participated?
How were the data collected?
How were the data analyzed?
What were the important findings?

Credibility Profile

Were all the important features of the main variable examined?
If there were several variables, was their selection well justified?
Were the variables of interest well defined? Is it clear how they were measured?
Are the participants (or respondents) representative of the target population? (Random sampling from the population and a high participation/response rate are the best assurances of representativeness.)
If a survey, was any attempt made to consider the issue of the extent to which the respondents resemble the target population?
If a survey, was the interview schedule or questionnaire thoughtfully constructed, pilot tested, and revised?
Were the data thoroughly analyzed?
How does this finding compare to other findings in the field?

OVERALL, IS THE FINDING CREDIBLE? Yes _____ No _____

Clinical Significance Profile

Do I think the incidence, prevalence, distribution, patterns, trends, and interrelations of variables are clinically meaningful in size and importance?
Are the differences between subgroups or between populations large enough to make a clinical difference?
Are the important results present in a large proportion of the participants/respondents?

IS THE FINDING CLINICALLY MEANINGFUL? Yes _____ No _____

Applicability Profile

To what groups of patients or situations can I extend the finding with confidence?
How effective is my current practice? On what rationale is my current practice based?
How *could* I change my practice based on this finding? Would this be a substantial, incremental, or soft change?
If I changed my practice in this way, could patients be subjected to potential harm, risk, or unreasonable effort?
Are there any organizational, logistical, cost, or time barriers to changing my practice? Could they be overcome?

SHOULD I CHANGE MY PRACTICE BASED ON THIS FINDING? Yes _____ No _____

How should I go about making the change?

Once I change my practice, how will I know if patients have benefited?

STUDIES USING NON-EXPERIMENTAL CORRELATIONAL DESIGNS

Understanding Correlational Designs

Many research questions are created to guide inquiry about the nature of relationships between or among variables. In this section several different types of designs will be discussed under the label correlational designs; the design type include descriptive correlational, predictive correlational, and model testing correlational designs. Descriptive correlational designs merely explore the strength of association between variables in a representative sample; one study of this type examined the relationships between psychological responses (anxiety and depression) and quality of life in patients undergoing autologous bone marrow transplantation (Gaston-Johansson and Foxall, 1996). Predictive correlational designs (also called regression model designs) explore the influence of one or more predictor variables on an outcome variable. An example of a study in which prediction was the main objective is a study of emotional distress reported by wives and husbands prior to breast biopsy (Northouse, Jeffs, Cracchiolo-Caraway, et al., 1995). Levels of social support, marital satisfaction, family functioning, hopelessness, concurrent stress, and uncertainty were studied as predictors of both wives' and husbands' distress; together these variables accounted for 42 percent of the variance in the wives' distress scores and 42 percent of the variance in the husbands' distress scores. Concurrent stress, lower education, hopelessness, and uncertainty explained the most variance in wives' distress, whereas concurrent stress, hopelessness, and family functioning explained the most variance in husbands' distress. Model testing correlational designs test the network of relationships among variables proposed by a theory or causal model. In a study of this type an explanatory model of nine variables influencing functional status in chronic obstructive pulmonary disease was tested (Weaver, Richmond, and Narsavage, 1997). In the sample of 104 patients, exercise capacity, dyspnea, and depressed mood directly influenced functional status, whereas dyspnea, depression and pulmonary function indirectly influenced functional status through exercise capacity; and self-esteem and anxiety indirectly influenced functional status through depressed mood.

As the above examples illustrate, a broad range of study designs fall into the category of non-experimental, correlational studies. However, all three types of study designs have in common the purpose of examining the relationships that exist between or among variables (Burns and Grove, 1997).

The appraisal questions provided for studies using correlational designs were developed to help you determine what kind of correlational study you are appraising, and will be useful even if you aren't sure about the type of correlational design you used. These questions will specifically and completely guide you in appraising descriptive correlational studies. However, the questions are less complete in regard to appraisal of predictive correlational studies and model testing correlational studies; these two types of studies are very complex and full appraisal of their scientific credibility requires advanced research knowledge. If you are uncertain about the characteristics of these three types of correlational designs or want to know more about them, you will undoubtedly find it helpful to refer to a research methods textbook. This increased knowledge will enable you to answer the appraisal questions more fully.

Many correlational studies are guided by trusted theories that help decide what variables to examine or help form hypotheses about the relationships between or among variables; theories also guide interpretation of the data. Other correlational studies test the web of relationships that have been proposed by a theory. Thus, theory is often prominent in the design, analysis, and interpretation stages of correlational studies as it provides an explanation for how, and sometimes for the mechanism by which, the variables are related.

Interpreting the Findings

Generally, descriptive correlational studies are very useful in studying the strength and pattern of relationships among variables, but care must be taken in interpreting the findings. First and foremost is the caveat that correlation between variables does not mean they are causally related. Causality is usually established through a series of experimental or quasi-experimental studies. Sometimes, however, a correlational design is the only feasible way of getting information about an issue and can provide valuable information that, when combined with findings from other non-experimental studies, can make a convincing case for causality. Second, the associations identified by establishing correlation may be much more intricate than what is suggested by the statistical data. There could for instance, be another unknown variable that influences both the variables that were found to be correlated, thus the two variables change in step with one another even though they don't influence one another.

Another concern exists with descriptive correlational studies examining many variables; if multiple correlation coefficients were calculated, there is a high probability that some of them may be statistically significant just by chance, i.e., the result of statistical "fishing." The report of such studies should indicate whether adjustments have been made for this likelihood (Type I error) and which correlations held up once the adjustments were made (Huck and Cormier, 1996). Often correlation coefficients that were significant before adjustment are not significant afterwards.

A final concern in interpreting the findings from a descriptive correlational study is that a correlation coefficient may be statistically significant, but is so low as to not have practical significance. As discussed in Chapter 7, the practical meaning of r is best understood by calculating the coefficient of determination, r^2.

Importance of Measuring Instruments

Since all types of correlational studies involve measuring several or many variables in a population or situation, the quality of the measuring instruments used is critical to the meaningfulness of the findings. The findings are much more credible if the measuring instruments have been tested and developed to ensure high reliability and validity. All research texts discuss these characteristics of measuring instruments, so you may want to reread that information.

In addition, to detect a statistically significant correlation it is important that a wide range of scores on the measuring instrument be represented by the sample scores (Burns and Grove, 1997); if the scores were within a very narrow range, it is possible that an actual correlation was overlooked, i.e., a false negative result was obtained. In the same vein, a data point located away from the bulk of the scores, i.e., an outlier, can distort the size of the correlation coefficient in either direction and may need to be removed prior to calculating the correlation coefficient (Huck and Cormier, 1996). When the report describes the range of scores represented and addresses whether there was a search for outliers, your confidence in the credibility of the findings should be bolstered.

Appraisal Questions

Synopsis

What was the general topic or question of interest?
What variables were studied?
Was the strength of relationship between variables examined, or were some used to predict others? Was a model composed of many variables tested?
What population does the sample represent?
How large was the sample?
What correlations/associations between variables were statistically significant?

Credibility Profile

Are the reasons for studying the variables plausible and/or connected to previous theoretical and/or empirical work in the field?

Were the research variables translated into measurements in logically sound ways?

Do the measuring instruments used have established reliability and validity?

Was the sample selected in a way that convinces me that it is representative of the target population?

Is the sample size large enough to detect associations (i.e., sufficient statistical power)?

If many correlations, or associations, were calculated, was there an adjustment to avoid chance results of significant correlations (Type I error)?

Were the sample's scores distributed across a wide range of possible scores on the measuring instrument?

Did the researcher indicate if there was a search for outliers and a thoughtful decision made regarding their inclusion in the computation of the correlation coefficient?

How does this finding compare to other findings in the field?

OVERALL, IS THE FINDING CREDIBLE? Yes _____ No _____

Clinical Significance Profile

In descriptive correlational studies, how strong is the association found between the variables? What is the amount of co-influence, i.e., what is the r^2 level? Does it indicate a strong or weak connection?

In predictive correlational studies, is the proportion of the outcome variable predicted by the independent variable(s) large enough to have practical meaning, i.e., what is the R^2 value? What variables have a large amount of influence on the outcome variable?

In model testing correlational studies, what proportion of the outcome variable is predicted by the other variables in the trimmed or revised model, i.e., what is its R^2 value? What pathways of influence are clinically important?

IS THE ASSOCIATION BETWEEN/AMONG VARIABLES CLINICALLY MEANINGFUL IN SIZE AND IMPORTANCE? Yes _____ No _____

Applicability Profile

To what groups of patients or situations can I extend this finding with confidence?

How *could* I change my practice based on this finding? Would this be a substantial, incremental, or soft change?

If I changed my practice in this way, would patients be subjected to potential harm or risk?

How effective is my current practice? On what rationale is my current practice based?

Are there any organizational, logistical, cost, or time barriers to changing my practice? How could they be overcome?

SHOULD I CHANGE MY PRACTICE BASED ON THIS FINDING? Yes _____ No _____

How should I go about making the change?
Once I change my practice, how will I know if patients have benefited?

STUDIES USING EXPERIMENTAL DESIGNS

Understanding Experimental Designs

There is wide agreement that when evaluating the effectiveness of a therapy or clinical intervention the most dependable evidence can be obtained from clinical experiments that (a) randomly assign participants to two or more treatment groups, (b) control the delivery of the treatment and the conditions under which it is delivered, (c) blind investigators and participants to which group a participant is in, (d) include patients who dropped out or didn't comply with the experimental protocol in the data analysis, and (e) have a sample size that is sufficient to detect a significant difference between the treatment groups.

When randomized experiments are conducted to test a clinical treatment's effectiveness using a large heterogeneous sample of patients, typically involving several data collection sites, they are called randomized clinical trials. Random assignment to treatment groups is of great importance because it distributes known and unknown extraneous, i.e., confounding, variables equally among the treatment groups, thereby assuring that the composition of the groups is unbiased. In randomized studies with small sample sizes, it is advisable for the researcher to compare demographic variables in the treatment groups as a way of checking to be sure that randomization actually did distribute known confounding variables evenly across the groups.

Controls put in place to assure that extraneous variables do not influence the outcome variable include assuring that the intervention is delivered in a consistent manner, that there is no cross-over influence from the treatment group to the control group, and that setting events that could influence the outcome variables don't occur (Cook and Campbell, 1979). The use of a control group enables the researcher to compare the performance of the treatment group(s) to a group who did not receive an intervention but was exposed to the same passage of time. Blinding of raters, care givers, and patients is important because it reduces biasing of perceptions or ways of acting on everyone's part (Dunn and Everitt, 1995).

The requirement of including all patients who entered the study in the data analysis rather than ignoring dropouts or those who didn't comply with the experimental treatment assures an accurate estimation of the effect of the treatment's effects (Jansen-McWilliams, Schwartz, Kalcevic, and Zeigler, 1996). This approach to analysis is based on the assumption that the reasons for not following a protocol, dropping out of a study, or not completing endpoint evaluations are important because they may have had something to do with a side effect of one of the treatments that could influence real-world treatment effectiveness (which the study-world should attempt to mirror).

Experimental studies require samples sufficient in size to assure that the clinical effectiveness of an intervention can be detected by the statistics used to compare the groups' outcomes. If the sample is too small, the study is described as lacking in statistical power, meaning the study has a low chance of confirming a difference between groups that really does exist. If the sample size is large enough for the statistics to detect a real difference, the study is described as having adequate statistical power. It is important that the researcher, in advance of doing an experimental or quasi-experimental study, conduct a power analysis to determine the sample size that was needed to have a certain chance (typically 80 percent) of detecting a significant difference if one actually does exist. If you are not knowledgeable about the concept of statistical power, you should read more about it in your research text, as it is an important characteristic of all studies using inferential statistics. To the extent that a clinical experiment lacks any of the five important characteristics just discussed, the evidence is less credible than evidence from a study that has all five characteristics.

The Potential for False Positive Findings

If a difference between treatment groups was a finding of the study, the appraiser should not accept this claim on face value; rather, she should ask if something about the way the study was done could have caused the difference rather than the experimental treatment *itself*. Original differences in the makeup of the groups as a hidden cause of differences in outcomes are more likely when randomization is not used. However, other hidden influences may still operate in randomized studies, including (a) the effect of special attention of the experimental treatment on the patient-participants of one of the groups; (b) resentful demoralization of those in the control group or less desirable treatment group; and (c) the effects of a pretest (or a posttest) in interaction with the experimental treatment (Cook and Campbell, 1979). Another design feature that can produce a false positive claim of subgroup or outcome differences is the use of too many subgroup comparisons or the use of too many dependent variables, resulting in a "statistical fishing" result (Cook and Campbell, 1979). In short, there are several aspects of conducting a study that can contribute to false positive results, and this possibility needs to be explored as part of appraising the credibility of the study's findings.

The Potential for False Negative Findings

A similar situation exists when no differences are found between treatment groups in a study. In this situation, the reviewer must ask if something about the way the study was done could have blurred the difference or resulted in failure to detect a difference that really was there. The most common design contributors to false negative results are (a) low statistical power; (b) lack of standardization in the way an experimental treatment was delivered; (c) cross-over influences between the patients and/or the clinicians in the treatment groups; (d) measuring instruments that were unreliable; and (e) reactivity by study participants to an intervention that was intended to be helpful but was experienced by the recipients as a burden (Cook and Campbell, 1979). Again, there are numerous reasons other than the ineffectiveness of the experimental treatment that could produce results that have an appearance of no difference in the outcomes of the treatment groups, but are really false negative results.

There are other features of a study that can produce either a false positive or a false negative result (Guyatt, Sackett, Cook and the Evidence-Based Medicine Working Group, 1993). For example, failure to take into account differential dropout rates between groups and failure to check to determine if patients complied with their treatment regimen can affect results in either direction. Another hidden influence that can systematically influence results in either direction is the unintentional influence of the clinicians and study assistants involved in the study; if they are aware of the treatment groups patients are in, i.e., they are not blinded, this could affect how they assess or rate patients on the outcomes of interest.

The critical issue in appraising the credibility of experimental and quasi-experimental studies is for the reviewer to deliberate over the question, "What else other than the effectiveness, or the ineffectiveness, of the experimental treatment could have produced these statistical results?" Although this skepticism is much more important for quasi-experimental studies, it should not be neglected when appraising experimental studies. Practitioners often have valuable insights to bring to the deliberation regarding possible confounding variables, because confounding involves clinical issues as much as it does research design. Ideally, the researcher has given thought to these issues also, and discussed them in the concluding section of the research report, sometimes under the subheading of limitations of the study.

Consideration of Individual Differences

Experimental designs examining possible interactions between an intervention and personal or contextual factors that may influence whether the intervention is effective or not are important to understanding how individual differences affect intervention effectiveness. For example, a study of the effect of home health care services on family caregivers' mental well-being found that on average the care did not make a difference in the strain and depression caregivers experience (Schwarz and Blixen, 1997). Further analysis, however, may reveal that family caregivers who have high burdens of care benefited a great deal from home care services, whereas care givers with low burdens benefited only a small amount; if this were the case, we would say that there is an interaction between the treatment and a caregiver's burden of care; that is, home care services have a differential benefit depending on the caregiver's burden of care.

Factorial designs, in which a treatment variable and a patient variable can be analyzed in interaction with one another, are a fairly common example of these more complicated types of designs. Unfortunately, studies examining these kinds of more complex relationships require sophisticated design and analysis techniques that can make the study difficult to comprehend. In spite of their complexity, the attempt to capture the dynamics of the real world rather than ignore the effects of individual differences is usually appreciated by clinicians because such studies are often in touch with clinical subtleties.

Clinical Significance and Applicability

When appraising the clinical significance of an intervention study, the measures of clinical significance described in Chapter 7 will be extremely useful. If the researcher did not report the data using one of the measures of clinical significance, you should calculate at least one of them yourself to gain a practical sense for the size of the difference between outcomes of the groups. The measures of clinical significance provide you with some sense of how large the effects of the treatment were and of how likely your patient is to realize a benefit.

Risk of harm most certainly should be factored into the judgment about whether to change your practice; therefore, it is important to note whether the treatment had any side effects or other undesirable sequelae such as inordinate burden on the patient or family or a high financial cost. The probability of adverse events occurring and the degree of burden can be taken into account using clinical logic or more formally by calculating a combined risk-benefit probability. Guyatt, Sackett, Cook, et al. (1994) explained how to calculate a risk-benefit ratio using the example of anticoagulation therapy for atrial fibrillation in which they calculated the number of bleeds per stroke prevented.

In addition to adverse events, you will want to take into consideration the effort, burden, financial cost, and other risks involved. If a rehabilitation program achieved its success at a very high financial cost or required additional long-term, in-patient care over what is involved in standard care, its effect would be viewed differently than if it achieved its outcomes with the same costs as standard care. The bottom line in the appraisal of the applicability of a treatment is whether the likely benefits are worth any potential harm, effort, and cost incurred—and these tradeoffs must be considered vis-à-vis nontreatment as well as other forms of treatment.

Then, of course, you ultimately are concerned with the question of whether a certain action will benefit a particular patient. The answer to this question rests on the size of the treatment's effect as well as the degree to which the patient is similar to those enrolled in the study or to a particular subgroup of the study. Often the total sample will be divided into subgroups based on age, gender, or any characteristic that might affect how they respond to the treatment, and each subgroup's data analyzed separately. Subgroup analysis has the potential to help in identifying differential responses to an intervention across subgroups; however, it also has great potential for misleading conclusions because it may take the form of "statistical fishing," which increases the chances of concluding that there is an effect when there really isn't. When considering the results of subgroup analyses, generally the size of differences among subgroups should be large, the difference should be statistically significant (preferably after adjustment for multiple tests), and the subgroup comparison should have been one of a small number tested (Oxman and Guyatt, 1992) for one to have confidence in different outcomes discovered in subgroup analyses. Subgroup differences not identified *a priori* should be "viewed as hypothesis generating exercises rather than as hypothesis testing" (Oxman and Guyatt, 1992, p. 81).

Appraisal Questions

Synopsis

What interventions, treatments, preventive services, or therapies were compared?
What outcomes were evaluated?
What populations were targeted?
How was the sample of participants acquired?
Were the participants truly randomly assigned to treatment groups?
What intervention delivery and data collection procedures were followed?
What measuring instruments were used? Do they have established validity and reliability?
What were the important findings?

Credibility Profile

Were providers, patients, and raters blind to the treatment each participant received?
If the treatment was administered over a lengthy period, were there checks to assure that it was consistently being administered in accordance with original specifications?

Were all participants who were originally randomized to a treatment group included in the data analysis? Were drop-out rates and failure to follow protocol rates reported and considered?

If differences were found

Could something other than the treatment variable have resulted in the groups having different outcomes?

Was there a check to determine if random assignment actually did evenly distribute confounding demographic and personal variables?

Other than the different treatments, were the groups treated equally?

If differences were found between subgroups, was the number of comparison tests done small in number or were the results adjusted for multiple tests?

If no differences were found

Could something in the way the study was done have resulted in the two groups having similar outcomes?

Was the sample large enough to detect a difference among the groups if one truly occurred, i.e., was a power analysis done to determine sample size?

Were the treatments themselves different enough to create a real difference in outcomes?

Is the association between the treatment and the outcome(s) plausible based on other available knowledge and information?

How does this finding compare to other work in the field?

OVERALL, IS THE FINDING CREDIBLE? Yes _____ No _____

Clinical Significance Profile

Note or calculate a measure of clinical significance for each result and deliberate on its clinical meaning.

IS THE FINDING CLINICALLY SIGNIFICANT? Yes _____ No _____

Applicability Profile

To what groups of patients or situations can I extend this finding with confidence?

Were there serious or annoying side effects?

Does the intervention subject the patient to any risks?

Was there inordinate effort required of the patients to use the experimental treatment?

How *could* I change my practice based on this finding? Would this be a substantial, incremental, or soft change?

If I changed my practice in this way, could patients be subjected to potential harm or risk?

How effective is my current practice? On what rationale is my current practice based?

Are there any organizational, logistical, cost, or time barriers to changing my practice? How could they be overcome?

SHOULD I CHANGE MY PRACTICE BASED ON THIS FINDING? Yes _____ No _____

How should I go about making the change?
Once I change my practice, how will I know if patients have benefited?

STUDIES USING QUASI-EXPERIMENTAL DESIGNS

Understanding Quasi-experimental Designs

Some studies that compare two or more courses of action are not able to (a) employ random assignment of participants to treatment groups or (b) manipulate the delivery of the intervention, hence they are called quasi-experimental designs (Cook and Campbell, 1979). Quasi-experimental designs may use one of the design features of true experiments, but their *failure to use both design features* undermines confidence in their findings. When appraising findings from studies that did not use random assignment or that did not have control over the delivery of the independent variable (the treatment or intervention), the appraiser must be keenly suspicious that confounding variables may have biased the findings.

Lack of Random Assignment

The function of random assignment is to distribute known and unknown variables so that the comparison groups are equivalent in all respects except in regard to which treatment they received. The comparison of nonequivalent or naturally existing groups, i.e., groups not formed by random assignment, may be misleading because the groups being compared may be different in ways other than having received different treatments. That is to say that there may be personal or circumstantial reasons behind why they received one treatment and not another, and those preexisting reasons may account for the differences found as much as, or more than, or in combination with, the fact that they received different treatments. The potential for unrecognized, preexisting differences greatly weakens any inferences we would like to make comparing the outcomes of the treatment groups.

An example of a study using naturally formed groups would be a prospective study comparing two different treatments for incontinence in elderly men used at two different sites: clinic Metro 1 and clinic Metro 2. The concern would be that the two clinics may be different in respects other than the fact that they use two different treatments for incontinence. They might see a different mix of elderly men, either in terms of overall health, ethnicity, or social and economic factors. Or they might have different screening criteria and referral mechanisms for getting men into the clinic, which could cause one study group to include only men with more advanced cases, whereas the other study group may include men with more moderate problems. These factors could make the two groups nonequivalent right at the start, irrespective of which treatment they receive, and could produce an appearance of success of one treatment over the other. Another possibility is that one clinic might provide a more attentive service than the other, which could work together with their treatment approach to determine their outcomes; thus, this example also illustrates how lack of control over the treatment variables can systematically influence the results.

A prospective cohort study is a quasi-experimental study that can be used to study general population groups with different exposures to health risks or different treatments by following them over time (D'Agostino and Kwan, 1995). This type of study is useful in determining the timing of events and various risk rates of outcomes of interest after a risk exposure. The concern, even when matching the groups on important confounding variables, is that the hypothesized cause or exposure that was the basis of the group assignment may be linked to a hidden confounder. In addition, follow-up is often problematic due to withdrawal and loss of participants over time.

Many research designs and techniques have been employed to control known difference in studies that cannot use random assignment, including matching designs, stratification, pretest-posttest designs, repeated treatment and withdrawal designs, propensity scores, and statistical adjustment for covariate differences. However, the concern regarding unrecognized difference (past or present) still lurks. Most commentators require that to have any degree of confidence in the findings of a nonrandomized comparison of therapies, the size of the observed difference in outcomes must be large, the difference between the groups on known confounding variables should be small, and the cause-effect relationship should be plausible based on other knowledge (Weiss, 1996). If all three criteria are met, it would be reasonable to judge the findings as credible.

Lack of Control Over the Treatment

Direct manipulation of the independent variable (i.e., the delivery and nondelivery of the intervention or treatment) and control over the conditions under which it is delivered assure consistency in the way the treatment variable is tested. This control is very important in assuring that each person in a treatment group has received the same form of what is being called "the treatment" and that provider "additives" (enhancements or detractors) have not been inadvertently attached to the treatment.

A commonly used design in which direct manipulation of the independent variable is absent is the case-control study. In these studies, cases in which the outcomes of interest have already occurred are identified. A control group is formed; it comprises persons who do not have the outcome of interest but are otherwise similar to the members of the case group. Then a retrospective, comparative investigation and analysis of their prior risk exposure or treatment differences is conducted (D'Agostino and Kwan, 1995). Clearly, the exposure or treatment variables are not under the direct control of the researcher, nor are persons randomly assigned to treatment groups. Case-control studies are often plagued by poor records and participants' limited recall of past events. This design is used when outcomes of interest occur only infrequently or when a long period of observation is needed between treatment and when the outcome of interest is likely to occur (e.g., in studying different ways of managing a chronic illness).

Together, randomization and manipulation of the treatment variable establish analytical and direct control over extraneous variables that could affect the outcomes of interest. Therefore, the major problem with the use of quasi-experimental designs is "distinguishing the effects that are due to the treatment from those that are due to uncontrolled extraneous variables" (Brink and Wood, 1989, p. 58). The appraisal questions in the credibility profile will guide you to think about the possibility of extraneous variables being present in the study you are appraising. Claims of an intervention's effectiveness based on a study using a quasi-experimental design, must be appraised with awareness that there is a high possibility that some aspect of the study's design may have produced an appearance of treatment effectiveness.

Appraisal Questions

Synopsis

What interventions, treatments, preventive services, or therapies were compared?
Was the intervention directly manipulated by the research team?
What form of intervention did the comparison group or control group receive?
What outcomes were evaluated?
What populations were targeted?
How were the participants assigned to treatment groups?
How long were the comparison groups followed?
What cause-and-effect relationships were hypothesized?
What are the findings?

Credibility Profile

Were providers, patients, and raters blind to the treatment each participant received?

If the treatment was administered over a lengthy period, were there checks to assure that it was consistently being administered in accordance with original specifications?

Were all participants who were originally randomized to a treatment group included in the data analysis? Were drop-out rates and failure to follow protocol rates reported and considered?

If differences were found

Could something other than the treatment variable have resulted in the groups having different outcomes?

Was there a check to determine if random assignment actually did evenly distribute confounding demographic and personal variables?

Other than the different treatments, were the groups treated equally?

If differences were found between subgroups, was the number of comparison tests done small in number or were the results adjusted for multiple tests?

If no differences were found

Could something in the way the study was done have resulted in the two groups having similar outcomes?

Was the sample large enough to detect a difference among the groups if one truly occurred, i.e., was a power analysis done to determine sample size?

Were the treatments themselves different enough to create a real difference in outcomes?

Is the association between the treatment and the outcome(s) plausible based on other available knowledge and information?

How does this finding compare to other work in the field?

OVERALL, IS THE FINDING CREDIBLE? Yes _____ No _____

Clinical Significance Profile

Note or calculate a measure of clinical significance for each finding and deliberate on its clinical meaning.

IS THE FINDING CLINICALLY SIGNIFICANT? Yes _____ No _____

Applicability Profile

To what groups of patients or situations can I extend this finding with confidence?

Were there serious or annoying side effects? Was there inordinate effort required of the patients to use the experimental treatment?

How *could* I change my practice based on this finding? Would this be a substantial, incremental, or soft change?

If I changed my practice in this way, could patients be subjected to potential harm or risk?

How effective is my current practice? On what rationale is my current practice based?

Are there any organizational, logistical, cost, or time barriers to changing my practice? How could they be overcome?

SHOULD I CHANGE MY PRACTICE BASED ON THIS FINDING? Yes _____ No _____

How should I go about making the change?
Once I change my practice, how will I know if patients have benefited?

SUMMARY

As the complexity of this chapter indicates, the appraisal of a single original research study is a multifaceted undertaking requiring an integration of clinical and methodological research knowledge. First you have to identify the type of study you are appraising and select the appropriate set of questions—at first, these two steps by themselves may be difficult. The reality is that it isn't always easy to determine what kind of study you are reading. Then it takes a while to learn to use the appraisal questions. Their meaning may not be clear at first or the importance of the issue they raise may elude you. Rereading the summary section about the particular type of study that precedes the appraisal questions for that type of study may help. Alternatively, rereading Chapter 7 may get you in touch with the broad issues in appraisal once again. The concepts of internal validity, threats to internal validity, and statistical power are critical to appraising the credibility of findings; therefore, you may find it valuable to reread these sections in your research texts.

The issue of clinical significance of results is an area of appraisal that is still in its infancy; still, some tools are available (e.g., ARR, NNT, difference in means, r^2). Health care researchers still have a great deal to learn about how to collect and present data so that the results of studies are useful to practitioners; they are still learning how to balance statistical inference and clinical significance in research reporting and how to blend the research perspective and the clinical perspective on knowledge.

The complexity of some of the material presented in this chapter may at first seem overwhelming to some readers. The reality is that to use research well, not just casually, requires precise thinking and awareness of the issues that can undermine the credibility and usefulness of findings. This doesn't mean that appraising research is so complex that only exceptionally bright people with a lot of time and research courses can acquire the skills. Rather, the knowledge of research methodology and the analytical skill required are considerable, and like any other complex skill, the ability to appraise a wide range of research studies is acquired one step at a time, over considerable time. Each time you read a study in an attempt to understand it, and use the appraisal questions, you will learn something new, an insight will creep (or flash) into view, and you will be one step further along.

You may be tempted to say, "I'm just going to rely on meta-analyses or integrative research reviews," but the catch is that the information from these summaries is only as credible as the studies included and as the methodology used to assemble and conduct the review. These summaries are typically much better at presenting their results than they are at explaining the strategic decisions that went into their analysis and conclusions. As more peer-reviewed meta-analyses and integrative review articles become available, and as the standards become more precise and demanding, you will undoubtedly be able to rely more on them. You should be aware, however, that they are not always the easy and dependable answer you (in your dreams) would like them to be. The credibility of their conclusions needs to be appraised just as the findings from a single study do.

References

Aday, L.A. (1996). *Designing and Conducting Health Surveys: A Comprehensive Guide,* 2nd ed. San Francisco: Jossey-Bass.

Brink, P.J., and Wood, M.J. (eds.) (1989). *Advanced Design in Nursing Research.* Newbury Park: Sage.

Burns, N., and Grove, S.K. (1997). *The Practice of Nursing Research: Conduct, Critique, and Utilization,* 3rd ed. Philadelphia: W.B. Saunders Co.

Cook, T.D., and Campbell, D.T. (1979). *Quasi-Experimentation: Design and Analysis Issues for Field Settings.* Boston: Houghton Mifflin.

D'Agostino, R.B., and Kwan, H. (1995). Measuring effectiveness: What to expect without a randomized control group. *Medical Care, 33*:AS95–AS106, supplement.

Dunn, G., and Everitt, B. (1995). *Clinical Biostatistics: An Introduction to Evidence-Based Medicine.* London: Edward Arnold.

Fowler, F.J. (1993). *Survey Research Methods,* 2nd ed. Newbury Park: Sage.

Gaston-Johansson, F., and Foxall, M. (1996). Psychological correlates of quality of life across the autologous bone marrow transplant experience. *Cancer Nursing, 19,* 170–176.

Guyatt, G.H., Sackett, D., and Cook, D.J. (1993). Users' guides to the medical literature: How to use an article about therapy of prevention; Are the results of the study valid? *Journal of the American Medical Association, 270*:2598–2601.

Guyatt, G.H., Sackett, D., and Cook, D.J. (1994). Users' guides to the medical literature: How to use an article about therapy of prevention; What were the results and will they help me in caring for my patients? *Journal of the American Medical Association, 271*:59–63.

Huck, S.W., and Cormier, W.H. (1996). *Reading Statistics and Research,* 2nd ed. New York: HarperCollins.

Jansen-McWilliams, L., Schwartz, F., Kalcevic, L.S., and Zeigler, C.M. (May 1996). *Analysis by Intention to Treat in Randomized Clinical Trials: A Survey of the Literature.* Paper presented at Seventeenth Annual Meeting of the Society for Clinical Trials. Pittsburgh, PA.

Kerlinger, F.N. (1986). *Foundations of Behavioral Research, 3rd ed.* New York: Holt, Rinehart & Winston.

Laupacis, A., et al. (1988). An assessment of clinically useful measures of the consequences of treatment. *New England Journal of Medicine, 318*:1728–1733.

Lincoln, Y.S., and Guba, E.G. (1985). *Naturalistic Inquiry.* Beverly Hills: Sage.

Munro, B.H. (1997). *Statistical Methods for Health Care Research, 3rd ed.* Philadelphia: Lippincott.

Northouse, L.L., Jeffs, M., Cracchiolo-Caraway, A., Lampman, L., and Dorris, G. (1995). Emotional distress reported by women and husbands prior to a breast biopsy. *Nursing Research, 44*:196–201.

Oxman, A.D., and Guyatt, G.H. (1992). A consumer's guide to subgroup analyses. *Annals of Internal Medicine, 116*:78–84.

Sackett, D.L., Richardson, W.S., Rosenberg, W., and Haynes, R.B. (1997). *Evidence-Based Medicine: How to Practice and Teach EBM.* New York: Churchill Livingstone.

Schwarz, K.A., and Blixen, C.E. (1997). Does home health care affect strain and depressive symptomatology for caregivers of impaired older adults? *Journal of Community Health Nursing, 14*:39–48.

Streubert, H.J., and Carpenter, D.J. (1995). *Qualitative Research in Nursing: Advancing the Humanistic Imperative.* Philadelphia: Lippincott.

Weaver, T., Richmond, T.S., and Narsavage, G.L. (1997). An explanatory model of functional status in chronic obstructive pulmonary disease. *Nursing Research, 46*, 26–31.

Weiss, C. (1980). Knowledge creep and decision accretion. *Knowledge: Creation, Diffusion, Utilization, 1*:381–404.

Weiss, N.S. (1996). *Clinical Epidemiology: The Study of the Outcome of Illness, 2nd ed.* New York: Oxford University Press.

Appraising
Collective Evidence

The pathway of research-based practice that involves appraising findings from two or more studies examines a broader base of knowledge than does examining the findings from a single study, but it also requires more time. The extra effort put forth, however, has the potential to provide a more trustworthy basis for changing practice, and for this reason collective evidence is recommended over a single study as a basis for a change in practice.

This pathway (see Figure 9–1) has a shared beginning with the single-study pathway in that the findings of each study bearing on your clinical questions must first be appraised individually to determine whether they are credible. Then all the credible findings are brought together and appraised as a collective body to decide which findings merit your confidence. The combining process, which requires organizational, analytical, and integrative skills, is best described as a synthesis, because you are producing a knowledge conclusion from the findings of the individual studies. Many aspects of the individual studies must be taken into account, including their purposes, methods, sample characteristics, how the intervention was delivered, and ways of measuring the outcomes, as well as the direction and size of the findings. The conclusion regarding which findings earn your confidence will also depend on characteristics of the collective body of evidence; characteristics such as the consistency of the findings, the number of studies with findings in the same direction, and the types of study designs that produced the findings should influence that decision. Once you have reached a judgment regarding the meaning of the entire body of evidence you still must decide whether the conclusions will be likely to hold up with a particu-

Pathways of Research-based Practice

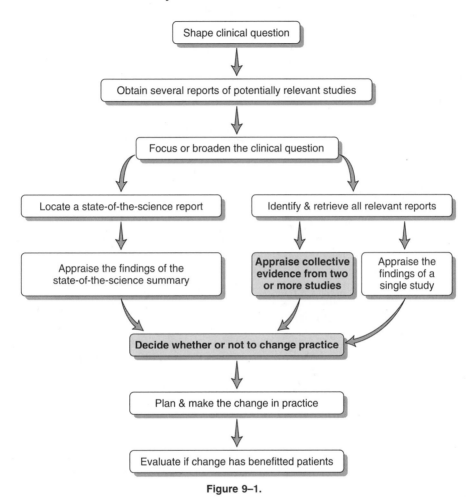

Shape clinical question

Obtain several reports of potentially relevant studies

Focus or broaden the clinical question

Locate a state-of-the-science report

Identify & retrieve all relevant reports

Appraise the findings of the state-of-the-science summary

Appraise collective evidence from two or more studies

Appraise the findings of a single study

Decide whether or not to change practice

Plan & make the change in practice

Evaluate if change has benefitted patients

Figure 9–1.

lar patient or with a population of patients. The complexity of this multistep undertaking should not be underestimated, for, as Cronenwett wisely observed, "Integrating research literature into a coherent argument for a practice innovation is no small task" (1993, p. 85).

The points of logic that enter into the appraisal of collective evidence are numerous and varied and have not been well explicated. Generally, the process of combining evidence across several studies could be described as across-studies synthesis, because the findings from each study become ingredients of a whole new knowledge product—your conclusion (or conclusions). The important thinking tasks of this synthesis include (a) considering the total body of evidence rather than favoring those studies consistent with your preferred thinking; (b) deciding whether to weigh evidence differentially based on study design or sample characteristics; (c) taking into account several different aspects of the total body of findings (e.g., consistency and sufficiency of the evidence); and (d) recognizing how your conclusions are determined by the studies you appraised as well as by the exclusion of those you didn't appraise (for whatever reasons).

In forming an overall judgment of the evidence, you will inevitably employ assumptions and inferences about the meaning and importance of each information bit; you should try to be aware of these aspects of your thinking, as they assuredly will shape your conclusions (Cooper, 1982). Assumptions are presumed truths that you don't think to question, whereas inferences are the conclusions you draw logically (the "therefores" of your thinking). If you are working in a group, you will have the advantage of being required to express your reasons for reaching certain conclusions about the evidence. A group process that works well will point out your assumptions and leaps of inference and verify their soundness or help you modify them to be more objective (i.e., less prone to individual bias). It may be helpful to note that the logic of appraising evidence across several or many studies is the same as that used by persons conducting an integrative research review. Before delving further into this chapter, you may want to revisit the sample collective findings table and appraisal of collective evidence provided in Appendixes F and G.

REDUCING THE SET

The standard regarding the inclusion and exclusion of studies to be appraised to answer a clinical question should be, as has been stated earlier, that all studies that directly bear on the question should be considered. An analysis of all six relevant reports on a topic might produce different conclusions than would an analysis that included just four of those studies. Although it may not be possible to appraise all relevant studies ("the set"), the method you use to reduce the set should be undertaken thoughtfully so as not to introduce bias. The decisions involved in reducing the set can slant the sample of studies you actually examine in ways that can change the nature of the evidence available to you. A sound approach would be to reframe your original question to focus on studies that directly pertain to patient end-point outcomes rather than also including studies in which intermediate outcomes[1] such as a laboratory value or an intention to enact a certain behavior were examined (Report of the U.S. Preventive Services Task Force, 1996). Examples of commonly studied end-point outcomes are functional activity, quality of life, death, and return to work.

If there is a large number of studies, the set could be reduced by

---

[1]See glossary for definitions of these terms.

considering only those conducted on samples of patients similar to those with whom you are considering using the results. If your question pertains to an intervention, you could reduce the set by including only those studies that randomly assigned participants to treatment groups. Other possibilities for objectively reducing the set include limiting the sample to studies published within a recent time frame, or randomly selecting from the entire set of studies a sample of studies that is of a size compatible with the resources you can devote to the project. Any partial use of all the studies available could influence your conclusions, but the approaches just mentioned should introduce the least bias for a specific purpose.

A common way of limiting the number of studies to be appraised is to rely only on reports found in journals that are at hand. Unfortunately, using the journal collection immediately available to you has a high potential to bias the set toward a certain type of study. For example, if only primary care journals were available, reports of larger clinical trials which typically get reported in prestigious specialty journals might not be included in the review, and this could be a serious omission. Thus, the best approach is to identify all relevant studies, then use one of the more objective methods described above to reduce the number you will appraise to a feasible number.

Fortunately, once an issue has received considerable attention in the research literature, the likelihood that an integrative research review or meta-analysis on the topic has been done increases, in which case you would be relieved of considerable work and often provided with a credible summary of the research on the topic. At this point, however, it will be assumed that you need to know how to appraise research evidence that comes from several studies. Before introducing the four sets of appraisal questions for collective evidence, some of the general issues that enter into considering a body of evidence will be discussed.

GENERAL ISSUES REGARDING EVIDENCE

Strong Evidence[2]

When appraising evidence from several studies, the ideal situation is when the research evidence is consistent across several credible studies as well as applicable to your setting and patients. Generally, you should consider *consistent evidence* from two or more studies as stronger than evidence from only one study. Findings across studies are considered consistent when the findings from all the studies examined point in the same direction, even though the size of the statistical result may vary from study to study. Findings

---

[2]The term strength of evidence refers to the quality, quantity, and pattern of evidence across several or many studies, not to the strength of evidence of a single study (unless that is all that is available).

are moderately consistent when the preponderance of findings are in one direction even though one or several are equivocal or in the opposite direction.

A group of studies with diverse findings or inconsistent findings presents a real dilemma, particularly when considering an intervention. In general, it can be said that inconsistent findings in any group of studies should be viewed with caution, and many factors must be taken into consideration when deciding whether to pick and choose from the findings. Among the factors to be considered are whether one or several of the studies are clearly better conducted than the others, whether any of the studies focus on patients similar to yours, and most important, whether any harm or risk would be imposed if you used the knowledge or therapy in question.

Types of Designs

In addition to considering the consistency and direction of the findings, the types of study designs that produced the findings should also be taken into account. Generally, a mix of designs on a topic provides a rich portrayal of a topic because each design contributes a different perspective on the topic. However, each type of design serves certain knowledge purposes better than others. If the goal is to understand patients' perceptions, a qualitative design is often the best design. If the goal is to understand a complex web of factors influencing a situation, a correlational design is most informative.

In contrast, when evaluating the effectiveness of an intervention the goal is to confirm a cause-and-effect relationship between the treatment and the outcomes. To achieve certainty about cause-and-effect relationships, study designs that control extraneous variables and control the delivery of the cause, i.e., the treatment, must be used. Therefore, it is generally agreed that a randomized experimental study provides more dependable evidence than a nonrandomized study, and that evidence from a single group before-and-after study, a cohort study; a matched case-controlled study; a single case experiment; or a time series study is more dependable than evidence from a correlational study. However, a series of correlational intervention studies with consistent findings can provide very strong evidence in support of, or against, a certain course of action.

Evidence from a *replication* study that validates findings from the first study is a very strong form of evidence because it confirms that the results of the first study hold up across time and different settings—that is, the findings are robust, not weakened by slight differences in application. Consistent evidence from two studies using *different research methods* is also a strong form of evidence because the findings have been confirmed from different perspectives and thus are likely to be independent of research methodology.

Composition of the Evidence

Your clinical questions will determine the types of designs and the range of subject matter of the studies you will be appraising. The most straightforward situation exists when your question involves an intervention. Even then, however, the body of literature will be intricate because of the following:

- There may be a mix of experimental, quasi-experimental, and correlational studies;
- Some studies may have used random assignment whereas others have not;
- The intervention may have been delivered differently in each of the studies;
- The outcomes evaluated may vary from study to study; or
- Several different ways of measuring the outcome may have been used.

The situation is even more intricate when the question involves an illness experience, a health behavior, a family response, or a rehabilitation trajectory, because the studies will be even more diverse in subject matter and design, making it difficult to compare and contrast them.

In Chapter 4 there was a discussion of how your clinical question determines the composition of evidence you will be appraising. The point was made that sometimes the evidence will directly bear on whether to enact a specific course of action, whereas with broader questions the evidence will consist of a collage or composite of evidence, each addressing a different aspect of the question. If you were able to focus your clinical question quite narrowly, the studies assembled may all directly address the same topic. Suppose the clinical question pertained to whether a particular technique for performing passive range of motion in persons with spasm of the upper extremities is better than traditional techniques, and the studies available compared several techniques for relaxation and stretching using experimental and quasi-experimental designs. The outcomes used in each study might be slightly different, but the studies would be quite homogeneous in design, and the findings would all directly address the question of whether the recently developed technique has any advantage over traditional techniques.

In dealing with questions of the type that lead to composite evidence (such as several aspects of taking an orthostatic blood pressure measurement as described in Chapter 4), it is best to group the studies by aspect, or sub-issue, and collectively appraise the collective evidence dealing with each sub-issue separately. In other words, appraise the studies addressing one sub-issue, set up a Collective Findings Table for just that aspect of the question, and then decide if there are consistent findings. Repeat the same process for each sub-issue. Clearly, you will have to appraise more studies than if your questions had been more narrowly stated, but by grouping them in terms of sub-issues, the collective appraisal will be more manageable. Some studies may have findings related to two or more sub-issues, in which case you would enter the findings relevant to each sub-issue on separate Collective

Findings Tables. In summary, you will need to be flexible and creative in the way you organize the display of your findings, as how you do it can facilitate your analysis or make it more difficult.

Clinical Significance

Appraising the clinical significance of the findings from a collection of studies involves transferring the methods used to appraise the clinical significance of the findings of a single study to multiple studies. Conclusions reached across studies must also be challenged in terms of their clinical significance just as individual studies are. However, the task is more difficult as the conclusions require combining the clinical significance appraisals of the findings from several individual studies; short of employing meta-analysis techniques, there is no convention for how to combine clinical significance information other than the use of comparative and integrative logic.

Logistics

When appraising the collective evidence pertaining to a clinical question, the studies assembled most likely will not all have the same design. For this reason the four sets of questions provided for appraising collective evidence are distinguished by the clinical topic on which they focus, not on the types of designs used as you did when choosing the best set of questions for appraising single studies. The four clinical topics for which a set of collective evidence questions is provided are (a) patients' experiences, (b) health or illness factors, (c) interventions, and (d) clinical assessment tools.

Studies of intervention effectiveness are a distinct topic grouping for which a set of questions specifically addressing how to collectively appraise the evidence for them can be offered. Studies examining patients' experiences and studies of health or illness factors each have unique aspects warranting a set of appraisal question for each topic. The clinical topic category of clinical assessment tools was added because practitioners often read about a measuring instrument or assessment tool that was used in research and wonder if it would be valuable to use in practice. Tools that have been developed and tested across several studies are most often preferable to ones that have only been tested in one study. In addition, these instrument development studies are quite different in language and design from other types of clinical research, requiring that a different set of appraisal questions be used to hone in on the

> **Collective Evidence
> Clinical Topics**
>
> - Patient experiences
> - Health or illness factors
> - Therapies and interventions
> - Potential assessment tools

important issues related to them. In summary, when appraising collective evidence you will need to select the set of appraisal questions from one of the four provided based on the main topic of your clinical question.

Earlier it was recommended that upon completing the appraisal of a finding that you found to be credible,[3] you complete a row of the Collective Findings Table which includes abbreviated information about the study, including author and date, variables or question studied, study design, sample size and profile, and findings. When entering the information from each study on this table you want to strike a balance between succinctness and a lot of detail. You want to have important information available, but you want to avoid being unable to detect it because it is lost among a multitude of information bits. With practice you will learn what is important to include and what is not, but a reasonable guideline at first is to limit the information to what will fit inside the boxes provided (after enlarging) using a moderate size script or font. An additional suggestion is that when recording the information on the Collective Findings Table you underline sample profiles that are similar to the patients whom you are considering using and findings that were judged to be clinically significant. An asterisk can be used to note findings that were statistically significant (i.e., don't bother with p levels or statistical values). Under the variables column, you should label independent or treatment variables (IV) and dependent or outcome variables (DV) if this differentiation is relevant. You may still have to refer back to your original appraisal sheets for needed information, but when thoughtfully completed the Collective Findings Table will assist you in identifying patterns and contradictions in the findings as well as differences among the studies that could account for the apparent contradictions.

Your Conclusions

Your conclusions will pertain to what findings you have confidence in after considering the total body of evidence. Like the credibility decisions you made regarding single studies, this conclusion will be the culmination of the answers to all the questions that have gone before it, and is a bottom-line judgment. The bottom-line question you will be asked to answer is: "What findings earn my confidence because they are well supported by the research evidence?" This question, however, is more complex than the bottom-line question for single studies because the number of factors you will be taking into account is greater and because you are required to recognize patterns and differences across studies.

---

[3]Studies that are so seriously flawed as to have dubious credibility, i.e., findings that have a high probability of bias or contamination from unwanted influences, provide tainted evidence that may lead to wrong clinical conclusions—and thus evidence from them should not enter into consideration.

APPRAISAL OF COLLECTIVE EVIDENCE REGARDING PATIENTS' EXPERIENCES

When examining evidence from studies regarding patients' experiences with health, transitions, or illnesses, you will probably be considering a mix of studies using qualitative, descriptive, comparative, and correlational designs. Some findings will consist of descriptions of an experience at one or several points in time, whereas others will portray the dynamics of an experience as it changes over time. Some findings will provide a deep description of one aspect of the experience, for example, how fatigue affects people's feelings about themselves, whereas other studies will describe the experience more broadly such as describing how chronic fatigue affects family relationships, work functioning, and the adaptive changes people have made to moderate these effects.

Your goal in appraising such studies is usually to *understand* what patients are experiencing rather than changing what you do, hence you will be considering a soft change in practice. Although the consequences of making a change in practice based on these kinds of studies carries the risk of misunderstandings and their effects on your relationship with patients, the consequences can usually be repaired if your change in practice turns out to be off-base. When considering whether to use findings from qualitative, descriptive, and correlational studies as a basis for a change in practice, it is particularly important that you pay attention to the profiles of the persons who constituted the samples so you can estimate to what extent their experiences will be like those of the patients you see.

One way of appraising evidence from several qualitative studies that may be useful for practitioners is to just not try to appraise them as an aggregate. Rather, recognize that qualitative research is a different way of constructing a picture of reality than is quantitative research. The fine-grained, often intimate, knowledge of an experience or of a social process that qualitative research conveys may not be amenable to integration across studies. Instead, qualitative research findings may provide us with a collection of different portrayals of an experience that is similar to the way we accumulate a repertoire of different patients' stories during practice. We don't try to homogenize them, rather we let each one reside in memory as a unique experience. And when a new situation resonates with a portrayal we have valued enough to save in memory for future use, the portrayal is activated and assists us in understanding what is going on in the present (Benner, 1984). In other words the integration occurs between a study's findings and similar real-life situations, not across qualitative studies.

Appraisal Questions

Across-Studies Syntheses

Note which findings describe the experience at a point in time and those which describe it over time.

Note which findings address the fine points or subtleties of an experience, and those that convey a better overall picture of the experience.

What findings are supported by more than one study?

Is there a compelling finding from just one study for an insight, factor, or association? Why do I consider it compelling?

What findings are outright contradictory from one study to another? Can these differences in findings be explained by differences in samples or research methods?

What findings resulted from studies using samples similar to the patient(s) with whom I will be using the findings?

Do any of the findings resonate with my experience more than others or provide a fresh view on the particular patient experience?

WHAT FINDINGS RELATED TO THIS PATIENT EXPERIENCE EARN MY CONFIDENCE BECAUSE THEY ARE WELL SUPPORTED BY THE RESEARCH EVIDENCE?

Change in Practice?

If I were to use the findings in which I have confidence, specifically what would I do differently?

Would making this change involve a substantial, incremental, or soft change?

Would inclusion of the finding(s) into practice impose any burden or risk on the patient, on me, or on the agency?

Would this inclusion be feasible practically and economically?

SHOULD I CHANGE MY PRACTICE BASED ON THIS FINDING? Yes _____ No _____

How should I go about making the change?

Once I change my practice, how will I know if patients have benefited?

APPRAISAL OF COLLECTIVE EVIDENCE REGARDING HEALTH OR ILLNESS FACTORS

Studies of the many factors and contexts affecting health and illness may use a wide variety of research designs including nonexperimental designs that are either descriptive, comparative, correlational, predictive, or model testing in purpose; and qualitative methodologies. This diversity makes it difficult to sort out the evidence because the studies often examine different combinations of variables from a variety of theoretical and methodological perspectives. For this reason, examining networks of factors associated with an event, behavior, or process is best done by employing a theory or conceptual model to bring the many factors together into an explanatory framework. Typically, there are many factors at work in a situation, be they family adaptation, individual coping, responses, events, onset or progression of disease, disability, health-related behaviors, or functional ability. Because of this complexity, it is often wiser and more practical to use a theory as a memory aide rather than trying to remember a market basket of unlinked factors. Thus, the across-studies appraisal of the factors and contexts of health and illness emphasizes the role of theory in putting together a complete and coherent understanding of a situation.

Thinking Tools

Using a theory is not imperative, but if a relevant one can be identified, it can be of great help in understanding a situation or behavior in which many factors or variables are being explored. If a useful theory does not exist, and even if it does, consider drawing a conceptual map that includes all the variables that have been studied and the relationships among them. An example of a conceptual map is provided in Figure 9–2. There are several variations on how to do this (Burns and Grove, 1997), but one approach is write down all the important variables/concepts that have been studied, grouping similar ones under or near one another and setting them up in temporal order from left to right if this is relevant. Then, underline the variables that have been found to be important and draw arrow lines indicating significant associations between variables that have been supported by at least one study. If an association has been supported by more than one study, darken the arrow with a bold pen or felt marker. If a theory that has been supported exists, draw a loop around the variables that are part of the theory. The somewhat messy map that results can be a helpful thinking tool, as it may reveal a clearer picture of the conceptual lay of the land and the empirical support that exists for relationships between variables.

Theory-in-Use

One item in the collective evidence set of questions asks you on what theory, or understanding, your current practice is based. You may have a tendency to say, "Oh, no theory, just experience, intuition, and common sense." But in fact over the years as you've accumulated clinical experiences with a certain population of patients, you have put together some explanation or way of thinking about their situation that helps you make sense of it, and this is "your theory" or your "theory-in-use" (Schon, 1983). It is your rationale for your current practice, and you need to evaluate new evidence regarding the context of health and illness vis-à-vis your current theory. Often when reviewing research on a familiar issue, you will slightly revise your current theory rather than totally abandon it. One practitioner working in a cardiac rehabilitation setting when first exposed to the Health Belief Model, realized that she rarely discussed barriers to enacting a new behavior and perceived self-efficacy to enact it with patients. The practitioner was impressed that the research evidence supported the importance of these two

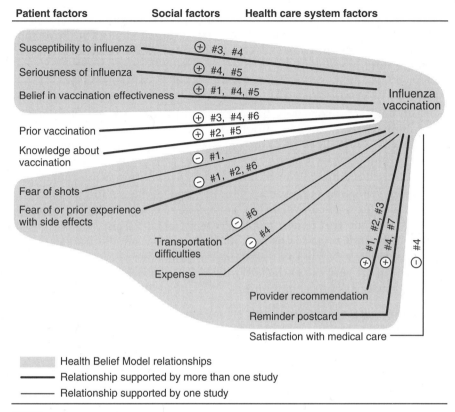

Patient factors   **Social factors**   **Health care system factors**

Susceptibility to influenza — (+) #3, #4

Seriousness of influenza — (+) #4, #5

Belief in vaccination effectiveness — (+) #1, #4, #5

(+) #3, #4, #6

Prior vaccination — (+) #2, #5

Knowledge about vaccination — (−) #1,

(−) #1, #2, #6

Fear of shots —

Fear of or prior experience with side effects —

Transportation difficulties (−) #6

(−) #4

Expense —

Influenza vaccination

#1, #2, #3
#4, #7
#4

(+) (+) (−)

Provider recommendation

Reminder postcard —

Satisfaction with medical care —

▨ Health Belief Model relationships

━━━ Relationship supported by more than one study

──── Relationship supported by one study

Studies

#1 Fieback & Viscoli, 1991
#2 Ganguly & Webster, 1995
#3 Gianino, Corazzini, Tseng, & Richardson, 1996
#4 Larsen, Olsen, Cole, & Shortell, 1979
#5 Nichol, MacDonald, & Hauge, 1996
#6 Nichol, Lofgren, & Gappinski, 1992
#7 Tucker & DeSimone, 1987

Figure 9–2. Conceptual map of factors affecting influenza vaccination in the elderly (based on data from seven studies).

elements of the model in helping patients adopt new behaviors. As a result, she changed her teaching approach to include these issues.

Appraisal Questions

Across-Studies Syntheses

What factors are supported as important by more than one study?

What relationships between factors are supported by more than one study?

Of the individual factor findings and relationship findings that were supported by more than one study, which ones did I consider clinically significant?

Is there a compelling finding from just one study for a factor, or association? Why do I consider it compelling?

What findings are inconsistent from one study to another?

What findings are outright contradictory from one study to another? Can these differences in findings be explained by differences in samples or research methods?

Is there a theory that explains how the factors work together to produce the behavior, situation, or process of interest? Do the findings support a particular theory that explains the experience, process, behavior, or situation? Does my conceptual map help make sense of the dynamics that bring about the behavior or situation or cause the process to play out in a certain way?

Were any of the studies conducted on a sample with characteristics similar to the patient(s) I have in mind?

WHAT FINDINGS ABOUT THIS SITUATION, BEHAVIOR, OR PROCESS EARN MY CONFIDENCE BECAUSE THEY ARE WELL SUPPORTED BY THE RESEARCH EVIDENCE?

Change in Practice?

On what theory or view of the experience, behavior, situation, or process is my current practice based? How does that basis compare to the theory or view the research evidence provides/supports?

If I were to use the findings in which I have confidence, specifically how would my practice be changed?

Would making this change involve a substantial, incremental, or soft change?

Would inclusion of the finding (s) into practice impose any burden or risk on the patient, on me, or on the agency?

Would this inclusion be feasible practically and economically?

SHOULD I CHANGE MY PRACTICE BASED ON THIS EVIDENCE? Yes _____ No _____

How should I go about making the change?

Once I change my practice, how will I know if patients have benefited?

APPRAISAL OF COLLECTIVE EVIDENCE REGARDING THERAPIES AND INTERVENTIONS

Appraising findings regarding interventions involves a particularly complex set of considerations. The research itself may be difficult to understand, and not infrequently, the evidence pertains to different outcomes or uses different measures of the same outcome. To be confident that an intervention is effective requires that the body of research establish a linkage between the intervention and the outcome. And to be confident about such a linkage, evidence from well-controlled studies is necessary. Added to these considerations about the research itself is the fact that the conclusion regarding the body of evidence may have ramifications for patient well-being, in that some degree of risk is frequently associated with health care interventions. To keep risk in perspective, it is often helpful to think about a particular patient rather than a population of patients, because the decision to use or not use an intervention supported by research ultimately must be made in light of each patient's unique set of circumstances and values. For that reason, the language of the collective evidence appraisal questions provided is framed in terms of making a decision regarding treatment of the individual patient.

Levels of Evidence

When appraising evidence regarding an intervention or therapy, it is widely recognized that a hierarchy of evidence based on the ability of the various designs to confirm cause-and-effect relationships should be taken into account. The highest level of evidence for establishing cause and effect between the intervention and the desired outcomes is findings from a multisite, randomized clinical trial or findings from several single site randomized clinical trials. A second level of evidence consists of findings from at least one quasi-experimental study, and the third is findings from a correlational or descriptive study. This hierarchy, displayed in Box 9–1, only addresses the effectiveness of the design of a single study in establishing cause and effect, and does not address the quality of the study or the overall strength of the collective body of evidence.

Although ranking of study designs by their effectiveness in confirming cause-and-effect relationships is appealing in its simplicity, the rigid use of such a ranking may lead to faulty conclusions about the evidence in that design flaws in any type of study can adversely affect the quality of evidence from any study, including those from a funded, randomized, multisite clinical trial. It also must be emphasized that each type of evidence can play a valuable role depending on the intervention being evaluated, and that results from several well-conducted quasi-experimental and correlational studies

---

Box 9–1

Levels of Evidence Regarding Interventions Using Design As the Criteria

Level 1
A multisite, randomized clinical trial or several single-site, randomized clinical studies

Level 2
A quasi-experimental study

Level 3
A correlational or descriptive study

can be as convincing as a single randomized clinical trial. Moreover, the findings of controlled experiments are often much more convincing if they are substantiated and complemented by the findings from well-conducted nonexperimental research.

Sufficiency of Evidence

In addition to considering the consistency of the findings and levels of design that produced the findings, you also need to consider the sufficiency of the evidence available. This is particularly important if you are considering an intervention and therapy that could put the patient at risk for an adverse consequence. You want to be sure that the evidence picture is complete, having addressed the following issues: potential harm or risk, benefits that have been realized, what types of patients benefited, what proportion of patients benefited, under what conditions of administration the intervention worked, and if possible the causal pathway by which the intervention achieves its benefit. This is to say that you would prefer that the evidence picture is complete, that there are no remaining unanswered questions or gaps in knowledge. Often, of course, one has to commit to a certain way of doing something without such a complete picture. You may want to reread the example on sufficiency of evidence that was presented in Chapter 2 (about exercise and breast cancer risk).

An important aspect of the sufficiency of the findings is whether the findings from the various studies have consistently been found to be clinically significant. Short of actually using the statistical techniques of meta-analysis, the most practical and useful approach to appraising clinical significance across studies may be to note this on your Collective Findings Table and take it into consideration in your across-studies evaluation. If three studies examined the effects of an intervention and all found an effect that was statistically significant but not clinically significant, you should surely question whether there is sufficient evidence to warrant a change in practice.

Inconsistent Evidence

When findings regarding a high-risk intervention are inconsistent, you should be very careful about using it. Although the variations in findings may be explained by the different methods, outcomes, or outcome measures used in the studies, the inconsistency may be an indicator of incomplete knowledge. Objectives in these ambiguous situations are to do no harm; to use the best evidence available; to not keep the patient from treatment that might be of known, albeit limited, value; and to reveal to the patient the uncertain state of available knowledge. One approach to resolving an inconsistent finding would be to call a person who did one of the studies with a positive finding, and ask if the patient with whom you are considering using the treatment falls into a subgroup that clearly benefited from the intervention. If that is not the case, the prudent course of action would be to not base your treatment on the research, instead to seek counsel from an expert or respected colleague or rely on your own clinical experience. A discussion with the patient regarding the lack of definitive evidence regarding a "best" treatment may help sort out the situation because some options may be more acceptable to the patient than others.

Low-Risk Interventions

When evaluating an intervention that involves low or negligible risk, the approach to across-studies appraisal can be less rigorous. For instance, the research evidence supporting the use of therapeutic touch or Reiki therapy can be less strong than what is required for prescribing a medication with serious side effects or an invasive procedure. The use of the energy therapies imposes no harm or risk to the patient whereas the medication does. The main potential harm associated with low-risk interventions is that patients will rely on them and abandon other therapies that have known efficacy.

The reality is that low-risk interventions are also less likely to be funded for large randomized clinical trials, so when you are considering the research base about them, you will often be appraising quasi-experimental studies and nonexperimental studies, all of which had small sample sizes because the researchers lacked the resources to use large sample sizes. As a result, you will be, and should be, skeptical in reaching conclusions about the effectiveness of the intervention. However, a small, well-conducted quasi-experimental or nonexperimental study may be very useful in providing early evidence regarding a potentially beneficial low-risk intervention—*even if* it did not have statistically significant results. One approach to dealing with inconclusive but promising findings regarding a low-risk intervention is to discuss the uncertainty with the patient and see if you can agree to proceed with close monitoring, frequent contact, and "how-is-it-going discussions." That way you may be able to combine evidence from your own clinical experience with the evidence from research in a way that uses a promising intervention yet does not put patients at risk.

Appraisal Questions

Across-Studies Syntheses

How much variation was there in how the intervention was delivered across the studies?

How much variation was there in the outcomes studied across the studies?

What findings are supported by more than one study?

What findings are supported by just one study but are compelling? Why are they compelling?

What findings are inconsistent across studies?

What findings are outright contradictory across studies?

Note the levels of evidence from the various studies and the findings associated with them. Is a randomized clinical trial feasible? Are findings from one available?

Of the consistent findings, how many studies had a treatment effect that was clinically significant?

What outcome(s) is this intervention highly effective in bringing about?

What side effects, harm, or burden is associated with this intervention?

Is the evidence picture sufficiently complete (i.e., knowledge regarding: benefits, risks, burden, underlying mechanism, specifics of administration)?

COMBINING CONSISTENCY OF FINDINGS ACROSS STUDIES, LEVELS OF EVIDENCE AVAILABLE, CLINICAL SIGNIFICANCE OF THE FINDINGS, AND SIMILARITY AND DIFFERENCES IN SAMPLES, IN WHAT FINDINGS CAN I HAVE CONFIDENCE?

Change in Practice?

Is my patient similar to those in whom the intervention was studied? Is my patient similar to any of the subgroups of patients for whom the intervention was beneficial?

Does my patient value the outcomes this intervention is likely to produce?

Is the intervention, including the burdens it imposes and any risks accompanying it, acceptable to my patient and me?

Do my patient and I possess the knowledge and skills to safely and effectively use this intervention? What would be required to acquire them?

Is the intervention paid for by the reimbursement system with which the patient and I are associated?

Would using this intervention involve a substantial, incremental, or soft change?

SHOULD I CHANGE MY PRACTICE BASED ON THIS EVIDENCE? Yes _____ No _____

How should I go about making the change?

Once I change my practice, how will I know if patients have benefited?

APPRAISAL OF COLLECTIVE EVIDENCE REGARDING POTENTIAL ASSESSMENT TOOLS

The phrase "clinical assessment tools" refers broadly to category schemes, rating scales, biophysiological measures, observational and interview schedules, and behavioral indexes that can be used to evaluate to what extent a characteristic or attribute is present in an individual. The attribute can be a health status; a functional status; a disease stage; self-care ability; a cognitive deficit; a health risk; a prognosis; a personality propensity; a physiological, emotional, or social state; a coping response; a behavioral intention; a quality of life index; or an illness impact. The Glascow Coma scale, the horizontal visual analogue scale for reporting pain intensity, and the Rhodes Index of Nausea and Vomiting are examples of such clinical assessment tools (Rhodes, Watson, Johnson, Madsen, and Beck, 1989).

Not infrequently, clinical assessment tools, or measurement instruments, are created in the research arena, but practitioners recognize their potential use and value for everyday practice. However, not all tools that work well in conducting research transfer well to clinical practice. The reasons are numerous: they may require special facilities or technically finicky equipment, take too long to administer, require the rater to be highly trained, or are not paid for by patients' reimbursement plans. In addition, many clinical measurement instruments are in the process of being developed and not enough is known about them to consider them reliable, valid, and discriminating. Also, the populations and conditions under which it is a valid measure, and population norms may not have been established.

Typically, when an instrument is being developed a series of studies are conducted to establish the quality of the data the instrument yields. These studies produce a body of evidence regarding the reliability, validity, sensitivity, and specificity of the instrument. In contrast, physiologic and physical measures are often described in terms of accuracy and precision[4] (Waltz, Strickland, and Lenz, 1991). The difficult issue for the practitioner is knowing when there is sufficient, supporting evidence to move the tool into use in the clinical arena. This decision, like many presented earlier, depends on both the strength of the evidence itself and on what constitutes current practice. If the current basis for evaluating a person's risk for elder abuse is very subjective, the practitioner may decide to use an index that is in the early stages of development in combination with the usual interviewing approach and criteria. On the other hand, one would hope that the instrument used to decide whether a person gets into a unique, costly, but very effective rehabilitation program would have had considerable testing, as a great deal hinges on the results. In one sense an instrument is never sufficiently tested because it will always need to be validated in each new population with which it is used, and our view of its reliability and validity may change with new knowledge, technological advances, or social change.

Evaluation of whether a measuring instrument is supported by enough

---

[4]To read an instrument development study and decide whether an instrument is ready for use in clinical practice, you need to understand these characteristics of measuring instruments. A definition of validity was provided in Chapter 6, and definitions of the others are provided in the glossary, but you will need to refer to research texts for a further discussion of them.

research findings to consider it sufficiently reliable, valid, and discriminating requires considerable knowledge of measurement principles. If you under-take an appraisal of the research evidence regarding a clinical tool or instrument, you will want to read your research text's chapter on measure-ment as well as the section on the particular kind of data instrument you are considering. Even then, it's highly likely that you will feel inadequate for the task at hand. You may have to settle for accepting someone else's appraisal of the evidence.

Valuable summary information about the instrument's reliability and validity status can be found in the introduction section and the discussion section of research reports about testing of an instrument. The researcher(s) undoubtedly has a better sense of the measurement issues in a particular field and a good sense of how a particular instrument performs in various situations. You will have to place some trust in the researcher and the journal that chose to publish the report as providing you with trustworthy interpretations and evaluations of the instrument. Another often very helpful action is to call the person who has been working on the development of the instrument. He may have new findings that haven't been published yet and may be able to answer some of your questions about how you would like to use the instrument.

Even though instrument quality studies are difficult to appraise, there are some things you can look for in a group of studies, and these will be highlighted in the across-studies appraisal questions. One of the important things is whether the developers of the study have been careful to be conceptually clear and consistent about what it was they were trying to measure. They should have started with a concept analysis or qualitative study to get a sense of the dimensions of the attribute or state they wanted to measure. They should be clear about what other concepts are similar to, but not identical to, the one they want to measure. Once the instrument was put together they should have conducted studies to confirm that it is accurately measuring what they thought it would measure. Ideally, it should have been tested in several settings and populations with whom it might be used. These broad steps, which are carried out in a variety of specific ways, assure that the instrument has been thoughtfully, methodically, and carefully developed.

Appraisal Questions

Across-Studies Syntheses

Specifically, what was the instrument designed to measure?
How carefully was the instrument developed conceptually?
How many studies have evaluated the reliability, validity, sensitivity, and specificity (or accuracy and precision) of this instrument?

What do the authors of these studies have to say about these qualities of the instrument?

Has the instrument been found to be capable of detecting small but clinically significant differences in patient status?

How many of these studies were conducted on samples and applications similar to how we will be using the instrument?

What risks or harms may be associated with the use of this instrument?

COMBINING CONSISTENCY OF FINDINGS ACROSS STUDIES, LEVELS OF EVIDENCE AVAILABLE, CLINICAL SIGNIFICANCE OF THE FINDINGS, AND SIMILARITY AND DIFFERENCES IN SAMPLES, CAN I HAVE CONFIDENCE THAT THIS INSTRUMENT PROVIDES QUALITY CLINICAL INFORMATION? Yes _____ No _____

Change in Practice?

How do I currently assess, evaluate, or measure the attribute this instrument measures?

In what ways am I dissatisfied with the current assessment tool/instrument?

How would adoption of the use of this instrument be an improvement over current practice?

In reading about how this instrument is used, can I see any reason why it might be unreliable, cumbersome, or difficult to use in our clinical setting (think of both patients and staff)?

Would adopting the instrument involve a substantial or incremental change?

Does my agency or practice have the resources to reliably use this instrument in an ongoing basis (i.e., equipment purchase and maintenance, personnel training, interpretation expertise)?

SHOULD I CHANGE MY PRACTICE BASED ON THIS EVIDENCE? Yes _____ No _____

Once I make the change in practice, how will I know if patients have benefited?

SUMMARY

The completion of a collective evidence appraisal and the resultant decisions about whether and how to change practice represent the culmination of a lengthy undertaking. It is undoubtedly clear to you why first searching for a published integrative research review or meta-analysis is the recommended pathway if you are limited in time. Still, the pathway involving assembling and appraising individual studies and then appraising the collective evidence can lead to insights into issues and access to a level of detail that is not possible using state-of-the-science summaries. Acquiring the skills to appraise collective evidence requires practice and time, but like so many rewarding activities, the more you do it the faster and better you will get at doing it.

References

Benner, P. (1984). *From Novice to Expert: Excellence and Power in Clinical Nursing Practice.* Menlo Park, CA: Addison-Wesley.

Burns, N., and Grove, S.K. (1997). *The Practice of Nursing Research: Conduct, Critique, and Utilization,* 3rd ed. Philadelphia: W.B. Saunders Co.

Cronenwett, L.R. (1993). Evaluating research findings for practice. *In* S.G. Funk, E.M. Tornquist, M.T. Champagne, et al. (eds). *Key Aspects of Chronic Illness: Hospital and Home* (pp. 79–89). New York: Springer.

Estabrooks, C.A., Field, P.A., and Morse, J.M. (1994). Aggregating qualitative findings: An approach to theory development. *Qualitative Health Research,* 4:503–511.

Report of the U.S. Preventive Services Task Force (1996). *Guide to Clinical Preventive Services,* 2nd ed. Baltimore: Williams & Wilkins.

Rhodes, V.A., Watson, P.M., Johnson, M.H., Madsen, R.W., and Beck, N.C. (1989). Postchemotherapy nausea and vomiting. *In* S.G. Funk, E.M. Tornquist, M.T. Champagne, et al. (eds). *Key Aspects of Comfort: Management of Pain, Fatigue, and Nausea* (pp. 243–258). New York: Springer.

Schon, D.A. (1983). *The Reflective Practitioner: How Professionals Think in Action.* New York: Basic Books.

Waltz, C.H., Strickland, O.L., and Lenz, E.R. (1991). *Measurement in Nursing Research,* 2nd ed. Philadelphia: Davis.

Studies Included in Conceptual Map

Fiebach, N.H., and Viscoli, C.M. (1991). Patient acceptance of influenza vaccination. *American Journal of Medicine,* 91:393–400.

Ganguly, R., and Webster, T.B. (1995). Influenza vaccination in the elderly. *Journal of Investigational Allergicology and Clinical Immunology,* 5:73–77.

Gianino, C.A., Corazzini, K., Tseng, W.T., and Richardson, J.P. (1996). Factors affecting influenza vaccination among attendees at a senior center. *Maryland Medical Journal,* 45:27–32.

Larson, E.B., Olsen, E., Cole, W., and Shortell, S. (1979). The relationship of health beliefs and a postcard reminder to influenza vaccination. *Journal of Family Practice,* 8:1207–1211.

Nichol, K.L., MacDonald, R., and Hauge, M. (1996). Factors associated with influenza and pneumococcal vaccination behaviors among high-risk adults. *Journal of General Internal Medicine,* 11:673–677.

Nichol, K.L., Lofgren, R.P., and Gapinski, J. (1992). Influenza vaccination. Knowledge, attitudes, and behavior among high-risk outpatients. *Archives of Internal Medicine,* 152:106–110.

Tucker, J.B., and DeSimone, J.P. (1987). Patient response to mail cues recommending influenza vaccine. *Family Medicine,* 19:209–212.

Appraising the Evidence from State-of-the-Science Summaries

When a body of research accumulates on a topic, experts in the field often bring the findings together into a cohesive summary that serves practitioners who are interested in the topic and researchers aiming to extend work on the topic. The results of several, or many, studies can be brought together in one of three summary forms: a meta-analysis, an integrative research review,[1] or a research-based guideline. All three forms are synthesized summaries because they produce new knowledge claims derived from the separate findings of the studies included in their analyses. These new knowledge claims should not be accepted on face value; rather, they should be appraised for scientific credibility just as any other finding is appraised.

It was recommended in an earlier chapter that when beginning your database search for studies to answer your clinical question you should first ascertain whether a state-of-the-science summary on the topic has been published. Following this pathway (see Figure 10–1) is particularly important if many studies relevant to the topic have been done, because basing practice on a state-of-the-science summary avoids the arduous work of locating, retrieving, and appraising findings from each study, and then collectively appraising them.

In this chapter the three forms of research summaries will be described, and important issues relevant to appraising each of them will be discussed;

---

[1]Integrative research reviews may also be called evidence reports, qualitative synthesis, and systematic reviews.

Pathways of Research-based Practice

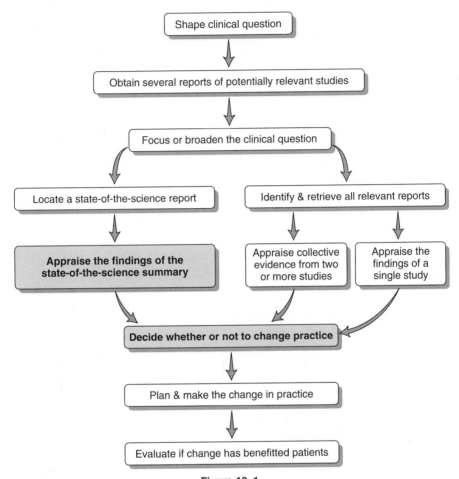

Figure 10–1.

a set of appraisal questions will be provided for each. In the meta-analysis section, the idea of treatment effect size and the statistics and measures used to represent it are introduced; this material will be easier to understand if you have a meta-analysis in hand to refer to. The same is true of having an integrative research review and a research-based clinical guideline when reading these other two sections.

DEFINITIONS

The meta-analysis (M-A) and integrative research review (IRR) both combine results from several or many studies, but the analysis and synthesis tools they use are different. Meta-analysis, also called quantitative synthesis, uses statistical techniques to combine results across studies, whereas an integrative review, relies on summations, logical synthesis, and narrative to characterize the overall findings. IRRs fill a middle ground between M-As and the traditional "literature review" in that they have a stated and specific purpose, follow a recognized procedure for constituting a sample of research reports (Cooper, 1982), display findings in tables that facilitate the identification of patterns and trends in the findings, and reach conclusions regarding the findings overall. Following all these steps clearly moves them to a level beyond the literature reviews reported at the beginning of research reports, which are often selective rather than being comprehensive and systematic as IRRs are.

SOURCES OF SUMMARIES

State-of-the-science summaries are available from a variety of sources. The best known in the United States are those that were published by the Agency for Health Care Policy and Research (AHCPR), which take the form of clinical practice guidelines and include the results of the M-A or IRR on which the recommendations were based. The clinical guidelines are quite specific and are accompanied by explicit indications of the amount of research evidence that exists for each practice recommendation. To continue helping practitioners stay abreast of the large number of research reports being published, the AHCPR in 1997 launched an initiative to establish a network of Evidence-Based Practice Research Centers to produce concise and clear syntheses of research evidence—this should result in the publication of even more high-quality research summaries and research-based clinical guidelines.

Another source of systematic reviews is the Cochrane Collaboration, which is an international organization that on a quarterly basis electronically publishes, on CD-ROM and via the Internet, high-quality systematic reviews of the effects of health care interventions and maintains a database of systematic reviews. The reviews and protocols of the Cochrane Collaboration are rigorously prepared and updated when important new studies become available. Their sites on the Internet,

http://cochrane.co.uk
and
http://hiru.mcmaster.ca/cochrane/default.htm

contain a great deal of information about the purposes and products of the Cochrane Collaboration as well as subscription information. The *Online Journal of Knowledge Synthesis for Nursing*, available through Sigma Theta Tau International, Inc., publishes critical reviews of research pertinent to clinical practice topics of interest to nurses in diverse arenas of practice. In addition, clinical and research journals of all health care disciplines and clinical specialities frequently publish state-of-the-science summaries on subjects of interest to their readers.

META-ANALYSIS

Although M-As and IRRs have been used mainly to evaluate the efficacy of interventions, both can be used to evaluate other clinical phenomena, such as the association between patients' risk factors and health outcomes or among contextual factors that influence health, illness, recovery, or adaptation (Reynolds, Timmerman, Anderson, and Stevenson, 1992). Generally, M-As are conducted when analysts think enough studies with sufficient commonality to provide a valid conclusion have been published, and when the analysts have the statistical expertise and resources to conduct an M-A. However, other factors, such as the nature of the studies and the nature of the clinical care in the area of practice, also influence whether a meta-analysis is done. The AHCPR panel that wrote the Clinical Practice Guidelines for Cardiac Rehabilitation (1995) elected not to commission an M-A because of the diverse, multifaceted nature of what is called cardiac rehabilitation, whereas the panel that wrote the Guidelines for Depression in Primary Care (1993) elected to do so.

Understanding the Results

When many studies on an intervention or group of interventions (e.g., health education methods) have been conducted but their findings are inconclusive, an M-A can provide a valuable overall perspective. By combining the results from the various studies, the statistical power of the new analysis is increased because the analysis is based on a larger sample than were the analyses from the separate smaller studies. As a result, meta-analysis often helps resolve issues about treatment effectiveness when a group of previous small studies have produced inconsistent or statistically insignificant results.

Treatment Effect Size

From the practitioner's perspective, meta-analyses can be difficult to read because a variety of statistics are used to quantify the effect of the treatment on the outcome or outcomes. Some of these statistics may not be familiar to the reader with basic statistical knowledge. Two features of *every M-A* are that an effect size is calculated for each finding included in the analysis (typically one per study), and a pooled effect size is calculated for all the findings together. Effect size is a statistical or numerical measure that quantifies the extent to which the treatment has had an impact on an outcome variable. Regardless of how the original researcher calculated the effect of the treatment, the person doing the M-A standardizes the statistic of effect size for each relevant finding using data provided in the original report, and then pools the individual effect size statistics to calculate an overall effect size. Thus, the effect size statistic or measure becomes a standard index, or common denominator if you prefer, that facilitates comparison of results from many studies and allows the results of all the studies to be pooled.

In a meta-analysis of studies related to whether oral antibiotics prevent infection in persons with dog bite wounds, eight randomized studies were found varying in sample size from 36 to 191 patients (Cummings, 1994). The relative risk (RR) of infection in patients treated with antibiotics compared with control patients was calculated for each study. The RRs varied from 0.22 to 2.11; some had very wide confidence intervals. The overall relative risk for patients treated with antibiotics was calculated to be 0.56 with a confidence interval of 0.38 to 0.82. This meta-analysis provided a more precise estimate of the benefits of oral antibiotics after a dog bite than did the previous studies individually, and also estimated that 14 patients must be treated with antibiotics to prevent one infection. Thus, this M-A revealed an overall trend in the results from the eight studies that would have been difficult to detect without such an analysis. Some researchers and practitioners consider a well-conducted meta-analysis of multiple well-designed, randomized clinical trials to be the strongest and most broadly applicable form of evidence available regarding a health care intervention.

Effect Size Statistics

There is an effect size statistic for every inferential statistic, but the easiest to understand is d. Effect size d has been used to standardize the size of the difference between the mean scores of two groups. It expresses in standard deviation units how far the data are from the null hypothesis being true, the null hypothesis being that there is no difference between the outcomes of the two groups. The value of d is the difference between the means divided by the common within-group standard deviation. Thus, the larger the value of d, the larger the difference between outcomes of the two treatment groups. The problem is that the value of d has little relation to clinical thinking—it has only statistical meaning. One way of making some clinical sense of an effect size index is to refer to the common interpretations of its values. In the case of d, 0.20 represents a small effect size, 0.50 represents a medium effect size, and 0.80 or higher represents a large effect size (Rosenthal and Rosnow, 1984).

Another effect size statistic, r, is widely used in meta-analyses. As a common index, effect size r accommodates results from studies with diverse designs and results that have been statistically analyzed in different ways (Reynolds, Timmerman, Anderson, and Stevenson, 1992; Rosenthal, 1991). The common interpretation of effect size r is that 0.10 represents a small effect size, 0.30 a medium effect size, and 0.50 a large effect size. Rosenthal and Rosnow (1984) prefer r over d in meta-analysis of intervention studies because r has a direct correspondence with the difference in treatment success rates found in a study. For example if the effect size r is found to be 0.30, there is a difference in success rates for the two treatments in the study of 30 percent, which is equivalent to increasing the success rate from 35 percent with the control treatment to 65 percent with the experimental treatment (Rosenthal, 1991). Thus, the value of r is identical to the difference in success rate (e.g., improvement rate, survival rate, gains in functional status); this, of course, makes interpretation of r easier than interpretation of other effect size statistics.

Measures of Effect Size

Fortunately, in recent years other measures have come into use in clinical meta-analysis as indexes to represent the effect of an intervention on a clinical outcome. The measures of clinical significance discussed in Chapter 7 (e.g., relative risk, success rate, improvement rate, numbers needed to treat) are increasingly being used as standardized measures of effect size in meta-analysis. Each of these measures provides a common index representing the treatment's effect on the outcome. The measure used in a particular M-A is usually chosen because it provides a clinically meaningful perspective on the benefits or risks of the intervention (Laupacis, Sackett, and Roberts, 1988).

To appreciate why different statistics and measures are used to represent the size of a treatment's effect on a patient outcome, you will have to read three or four M-As that use different effect size statistics and measures. The essential point, however, is that in *all meta-analyses* a statistic or a measure of effect size is used to represent the size of the treatment's impact on the outcome or the size of the association between two variables. That statistic or measure is calculated for every finding and then for all the findings together; often effect size measures or statistics are also calculated for subgroups of the findings that share the same outcome variable or the same form of the intervention. From the practitioner's perspective, the measures of effect size are preferable to the effect size statistics because they represent the effect of a treatment or risk factor on patient outcomes in clinically relevant terms.

Examples

A list of published M-As is provided in Table 10–1. As can be seen, the range of topics on which M-As have been done is broad, and the measures and statistics used to index the effect size varies.

Table 10–1. **Examples of Meta-Analyses**

Study	Treatment or Risk Factor of Interest	Outcomes of Interest	Measure or Statistic Used to Index the Effect Size
Psaty et al. (1997)	Antihypertensive therapies	Safety and efficacy	Relative risk
Brown and Grimes (1993)	Advanced practice nurse care versus MD care	Clinical outcomes, cost	Effect size (d)
Warshafsky, Kramer, and Sivak (1993)	Oral garlic supplementation	Total serum cholesterol	Difference in the change of cholesterol level (mmol/dL)
Smith et al. (1992)	Respiratory muscle training	Pulmonary function, respiratory muscle strength, functional exercise capacity, functional status	Effect size (d)
AHCPR (1993)	Treatment of major depression in primary care	Symptoms, interpersonal and occupational functioning	Difference in response rate
McCaul et al. (1996)	Risk of breast cancer	Having a mammogram done	Effect size (r)

Selected results from an M-A examining the relationship between breast cancer risk and mammography screening are presented in Table 10–2 (McCaul, Branstetter, Schroeder, and Glasgow, 1996). There has been some debate about whether women who are at risk for breast cancer are more or less likely to have mammograms done, and the rationale for each point of view is cogent; results of studies that included at least one of four predictor

Table 10–2. **Summary of Meta-Analysis of Breast Cancer Risk and Mammography Screening (from McCaul et al.)**

Risk Measure	Number of Studies in Analysis	Average Weighted Effect Size (r)
Family history of breast cancer	19	0.27
Perceived vulnerability to breast cancer	19	0.16
Breast problems	10	0.30
Worried about breast cancer	6	0.14

variables of mammography were included in this analysis. The analysts note, "For the two measures studied most frequently—a family history of breast cancer and perceived vulnerability—35 of 38 studies reported a positive effect between measures of risk and screening behavior" (p. 427), and concluded that risk has a small to moderate positive relationship[2] with screening behavior. They further opined that in light of the fact that having or not having a mammogram is so influenced by provider recommendation, the association between risk and having a mammogram, even though modest in size, is a clinically important one.

Data Presentation

Not only do M-As vary greatly in what effect size statistic or measure they use, they also use a wide variety of methods for presenting the data. Some use tables that consist of point estimates of effect size for the studies in the analysis; 95 percent confidence intervals around the point estimate of the effect size statistic or measure may or may not be displayed. Others graphically display the point estimates and confidence intervals in a way that reveals how much overlap exists in the findings from the studies. This is particularly useful if the scale indicates what is considered to be a clinically meaningful value on the effect size scale. Wide confidence intervals mean that the point estimate is imprecise, whereas narrow confidence intervals mean that the point estimate is precise. Small samples produce more sampling error and hence wider, less precise, confidence intervals than do large samples.

To appreciate the value of confidence interval displays, consider results from a meta-analysis of 18 long-term, placebo-controlled, randomized trials of health outcomes associated with first-line antihypertensive therapies[3] (Psaty et al., 1997). The four therapies compared were (1) high-dose diuretics, (2) low-dose diuretics, (3) beta-blockers, and (4) a Hypertension Detection and Follow-up Program (HDFP) which compared a diuretic-based stepped-care therapy to routine community-based referred care (rather than placebo). Confidence intervals around the effect size measure of relative risk (RR) for five outcomes (stroke, coronary artery disease, congestive heart failure, total mortality, and cardiovascular mortality) are displayed in Table 10–3. A relative risk of 1.0 would mean that the therapy was equivalent in

---

[2]A treatment effect of magnitude $r = 0.27$, as was found between family history of breast cancer and having a mammogram, corresponds to a difference in behavior of 27 percent between those who have a family history and those who do not (Rosenthal and Rosnow, 1984, p. 210). This additional interpretation of r adds important practical information to the deliberation over whether this effect size is clinically significant.

[3]The authors concluded that this evidence provides strong support for the use of diuretics and beta-blockers as first line agents until the results of large long-term clinical trials evaluating the effects of calcium-channel blockers and angiotensin-converting enzyme (ACE) inhibitors are available.

Table 10–3. **Results of Meta-Analysis of Antihypertension Therapy**

Outcome Drug Regimen	Dose	No. of Trials	Events, Active Treatment/Control	RR (95% CI)	RR (95% CI)
Stroke					
Diuretics	High	9	88/232	0.49 (0.39–0.62)	
Diuretics	Low	4	191/347	0.66 (0.55–0.78)	
β-Blockers	High	4	147/335	0.71 (0.59–0.86)	
HDFP	High	1	102/158	0.64 (0.50–0.82)	
Coronary Heart Disease					
Diuretics	High	11	211/331	0.99 (0.83–1.18)	
Diuretics	Low	4	215/363	0.72 (0.61–0.85)	
β-Blockers	High	4	243/459	0.93 (0.80–1.09)	
HDFP	High	1	171/189	0.90 (0.73–1.10)	
Congestive Heart Failure					
Diuretics	High	9	6/35	0.17 (0.07–0.41)	
Diuretics	Low	3	81/134	0.58 (0.44–0.76)	
β-Blockers		2	41/175	0.58 (0.40–0.84)	

RR (95% CI)

0.4   0.7   1.0

Treatment→ Treatment Better→

Treatment→ Treatment Worse→

				RR (95% CI)
Total Mortality				
Diuretics	High	11	224/382	0.88 (0.75–1.03)
Diuretics	Low	4	514/713	0.90 (0.81–0.99)
β-Blockers	High	4	383/700	0.95 (0.84–1.07)
HDFP	High	1	349/419	0.83 (0.72–0.95)
Cardiovascular Mortality				
Diuretics	High	11	124/230	0.78 (0.62–0.97)
Diuretics	Low	4	237/390	0.76 (0.65–0.89)
β-Blockers	High	4	214/410	0.89 (0.76–1.05)
HDFP	High	1	195/240	0.81 (0.67–0.97)

Meta-analysis of randomized, placebo-controlled clinical trials in hypertension according to first-line treatment strategy. Trials indicate number of trials with at least 1 end point of interest. RR indicates relative risk; CI, confidence interval; and HDFP, Hypertension Detection and Follow-up Program Study (5484 subjects in stepped care and 5455 in referred care). For these comparisons, the numbers of participants randomized to active therapy and placebo were 7768 and 12,075 for high-dose diuretic therapy; 4305 and 5116 for low-dose diuretic therapy; and 6736 and 12,147 for β-blocker therapy. Because the placebo group is included twice in these totals, once for a diuretic comparison and again for a β-blocker comparison. The total number of participants randomized to active therapy and control therapy were 24,294 and 23,926, respectively.

Source: From Psaty, B.M., et al. (1997). *Journal of American Medical Association, 277:*742.

effect to a placebo in preventing the outcome; thus, it is marked as a clinically meaningful point on the effect size scale of the table.

Among the results are the findings that when compared to placebo therapy, high-dose diuretics were effective in preventing stroke (RR = 0.49) based on the combined results of nine studies, and low-dose diuretics were effective in preventing coronary artery disease (RR = 0.72) and congestive heart failure (RR = 0.58). Beta-blockers were effective in preventing congestive heart failure (RR = 0.58) based on the results of two studies and stroke (RR = 0.71) based on four studies. Any group of studies with RR confidence intervals that do not include or extend above 1.0 found the particular therapy to be more effective than a placebo with that particular outcome; this was the case for 12 therapy-outcome combinations, but not true for six therapy-outcome combinations. You can see that this type of display conveys a great deal of information in an easy to use format.

Value of Findings

Although controversy accompanies the statistical techniques and assumptions of M-A, many experts view it as an objective analytic technique that has the potential to reveal intervention effect and association between variables that are not evident when logically comparing the findings of a group of individual studies (Cooper and Hedges, 1994; Devine, 1990; Cook, Mulrow, and Haynes, 1997). One investigation showed that the results of pooled data from smaller trials are usually compatible with the results of larger trials, particularly when differences in target populations and variability of treatments are taken into account (Cappelleri et al., 1996). Still, the practitioner needs to keep in mind that the overall estimate of treatment effect that results from an M-A may obscure findings from a particular trial in which the participants are like the patient(s) you are treating.

Appraisal Issues

Bias

Even though the methodology of M-A is not examined in most research courses and may be unfamiliar to many practitioners, some attempt to determine whether the M-A itself was well conducted must be made. There are several points at which bias can enter the analysis, and detract from the credibility of the findings. One of these points is when individual studies were selected to be included in the analysis; this is a crucial step in the analysis because the selection of studies itself can introduce bias into the M-A findings, just as the sample selection in a research study can. The ideal is that (a) there was a comprehensive and explicit strategy for locating relevant reports; (b) an explicit criteria for inclusion or exclusion of studies were used; and (c) the inclusion/exclusion criteria were consistently applied. Adherence to these standards assures that all relevant and well-conducted studies on the issue were considered when reaching conclusions about the intervention.

Although it makes sense to eliminate methodologically poor studies, the elimination of "poor" studies is another point at which bias can enter the analysis, because methodological evaluation is a subjective activity. Steps that should be taken to control bias when eliminating methodologically weak studies include (1) the use of an objective scoring method for assessing quality (Brown, 1991), (2) having more than one rater, (3) requiring that the raters be trained in using the scoring system and have attained a high degree of agreement in quality decisions, and (4) blinding raters to the names and affiliated institutions of the investigators who authored the report. In summary, there should be provision for eliminating seriously flawed studies from the analysis, but there should be evidence in the report that this was done with care to avoid the bias such a judgment can introduce.

Data Pooling Procedures

One of the issues involved in conducting an M-A is what kind of studies can/should be pooled for the analysis. The concern is whether the studies included in the analysis are similar enough in design, sample size, outcome types, and form of the independent variable to be pooled (Sacks et al., 1987). There are several ways this concern can be handled, and all are a bit difficult to understand. At the very least, the issue should be discussed by the meta-analyst; beyond that, a "homogeneity analysis" may be done or the confidence profile method of analysis which adjusts for differences may be used (Eddy and Hasselblad, 1994).[4] Although the practitioner is likely to have difficulty understanding the methodological discussions of heterogeneity of the studies, the inclusion of this consideration in the report reflects methodological rigor in the conduct of the analysis.

The analyst should also run the analyses with several different inclusion criteria and assumptions, e.g., with and without nonrandomized studies, with and without a study that has contradictory results, with and without studies of lower quality. These types of comparisons reveal how resistant the results of the M-A is to different ways of conducting the analysis.

---

[4]The confidence profile method is a collection of sophisticated statistical techniques for estimating a treatment effect by combining results of multiple studies. The treatment effect is adjusted for potential biases to internal and external validity and for differences in design and outcome types. The results of the analyses are in the form of probability distributions or confidence intervals for the parameters of interest (Eddy and Hasselblad, 1994).

Clinical Significance

Ironically, appraising the clinical significance of an M-A of a class of interventions is frequently more straightforward than appraising the clinical significance of a single study. This is because a table displaying the chosen measure of effect size for all the studies under review is often provided, and an overall measure of effect size is calculated. Many M-As are conducted to reach conclusions that will serve as guidelines for clinical practice; as a result, the clinical significance of quantitative summaries are often explicit in the way the review question is framed, in the way the results are presented, as well as in the discussion of the results.

Appraisal Process

The practitioner reading a meta-analysis report ultimately wants to know if an intervention has enough benefit that it should be used in practice. To determine this you must first get a sense of what question was being asked in the analysis, particularly what intervention or category of interventions was being evaluated and what it was being compared to. Then, you should attempt to understand how the M-A was conducted, which includes the characteristics of the studies included (e.g., research designs, participants' characteristics, outcomes of the studies, and specific measures used), as well as the common measure of effect size that was used. The next step is to appraise the credibility of the meta-analysts' conclusions, which involves challenging the scientific soundness of the meta-analysts' methodology (admittedly difficult for the novice appraiser). Finally, you should judge whether the intervention's effect would be likely to make important differences with the patients, or patient, you are treating. Toward the goal of making a good appraisal decision about an M-A, questions are offered using the headings that were used for the appraisal of single, original studies (i.e., synopsis, credibility profile, clinical significance, and applicability profile).

Appraisal Questions

Synopsis

What was the question the meta-analysis set out to answer? What types or classes of interventions were compared? What outcomes were studied? What associations between variables were of interest?
How were potential, relevant research reports identified?
What determined if a research report was included in the analysis or not?
How many studies were included in each part of the analysis?
What mix of design types was used in the individual studies?

What measure of effect size was used, e.g., an effect size statistic, treatment response rate, relative risk, numbers needed to treat?

What were the important findings?

What were the analysts' conclusions?

Credibility Profile

Was the research question clear and clinically meaningful?

Were the methods of the analysis reported in sufficient detail to enable a replication of the analysis?

Was the search for potential reports broad and unbiased?

Were inclusion or exclusion criteria explicitly set forth?

Was the credibility, i.e., scientific soundness, of the individual studies assessed? Was this decision made in a reliable and objective manner? Were seriously flawed studies eliminated from the analysis or analyzed separately?

Was separate information provided for randomized and nonrandomized studies?

ARE THE FINDINGS CREDIBLE? Yes _____ No _____

Clinical Significance

How consistent were the results across studies, i.e., what percentage showed a treatment effect in the same direction? If quite variable, could the differences be explained by differences in populations, treatments, or outcomes?

Was there a clear, consistently found result regarding the efficacy of a particular treatment, either when compared to a placebo treatment or when compared to another treatment? Was a relationship between variables consistently found?

Was the overall effect size large, modest, or small? Was the effect size clinically meaningful?

Was the effect size for any subgroup of studies of interest to me large, modest, or small?

DO I THINK THE ASSOCIATION BETWEEN THE TREATMENT OR RISK FACTOR AND THE OUTCOME(S) IS LARGE ENOUGH TO MAKE A DIFFERENCE IN PATIENTS' WELL-BEING? Yes _____ No _____

Applicability Profile

Are the resulting benefits of the treatment/risk factor impressive vis-à-vis the risks and cost?

Are the outcomes achieved of value to my patient(s)?

Are the patients I treat, or the patient I am treating, similar to any of those included in the analysis?

Am I able to safely and effectively use this intervention?

Are there any organizational, logistical, financial, or time barriers to incorporating this intervention into my practice? How could they be overcome?

What changes, additions, training or purchases would be needed to start using this intervention?

SHOULD I CHANGE MY PRACTICE BASED ON THESE FINDINGS? Yes _____ No _____

Once I change my practice, how will I know if the change has improved the care I give?

APPRAISAL OF AN INTEGRATIVE RESEARCH REVIEW

Integrative research reviews employ the same question asking, searching, and sampling techniques at the front end as do M-As, but when it comes to analyzing the results, they rely on logical comparison and synthesis, rather than statistical synthesis, to reach conclusions. To assure reproducibility of the results, an IRR should display the features of the studies analyzed in tables so the reader can see the raw, albeit condensed, data. Typically, these displays include columns for the reference and country where conducted, a brief description of the sample, a brief description of the intervention(s), outcomes and follow-up intervals, and the results of the study.

Explicit Rules of Inference

The rules of inference by which the results of the various studies were synthesized into an overall conclusion should be explicitly stated. For example, if more reliance was placed on the results of randomized studies, this should be stated, or if the analyst discounted the findings of a particular study for some reason, this should be acknowledged. In logical synthesis, the concern is that some sort of thinking or values bias may have influenced the analyst's thinking. By displaying the features of the individual studies in a table and by setting forth the rules of evidence invoked in the analysis, the analyst provides the reader with information on which to appraise the credibility of the conclusions. If this information is not provided, the reader is placed in the position of trusting the analyst's interpretation of the evidence, which is not in keeping with the explicit nature of scientific decision making.

Deep Comparison and Synthesis

There should also be an indication that the analyst compared the features of all the studies to try to account for disparate findings. Often the use of different patient samples, outcomes, outcomes measures (i.e., instruments), and measurement intervals, or variation in the way the treatment was delivered in the studies, can account for the different results. In short, one should get the sense that the analyst considered several different explanations for the findings and reached conclusions that demonstrated deep comparison and synthesis of all the findings in the analysis. The example appraisal provided in Appendix H illustrates the kinds of issues that should be taken into consideration when appraising an integrative research review.

Appraisal Questions

Synopsis

What topic or question did the integrative review address?
How were potential, relevant research reports identified?
What determined if a research report was included in the analysis or not?
How many studies were included in the analysis?
What research methods were used in the studies included in the analysis?
What were the important and consistent findings?
What were the analyst's conclusions?

Credibility Profile

Was the topic clearly defined and clinically meaningful?
Was the search for potential reports broad and unbiased?
Were the characteristics of the studies displayed or discussed in sufficient detail?
Is there truly an integration/synthesis of findings or merely a reporting of separate findings?
Do the overall findings accurately reflect the findings from all the individual studies?
What overall findings were consistently well supported and which were less well supported? What, if anything, could explain differences in results from study to study?

ARE THE CONCLUSIONS OF THE INTEGRATION CREDIBLE? Yes _____ No _____

Clinical Significance

Do the conclusions resonate with what I see in everyday practice?

WHAT FINDINGS ARE SIZABLE ENOUGH, CONSISTENT ENOUGH, AND WELL ENOUGH SUPPORTED THAT THE CONCLUSIONS ARE LIKELY TO HOLD UP IN EVERYDAY PRACTICE?

Applicability Profile

Are my patients similar to any of those studied? Are they similar to those in a particular study? Was there anything of note in the results for samples or subsamples that are most like my patient(s)?

Are the outcomes achieved of value to me or my patient(s)?

What were the key features of the approach or intervention?

Am I able to safely and effectively use the approach or intervention described?

Are the findings and conclusions impressive enough to warrant trying them in my practice?

Are there any organizational, logistical, cost, or time barriers to incorporating this approach into my practice? Could they be overcome?

What changes, additions, training, or purchases would be needed to start using this approach?

SHOULD I CHANGE MY PRACTICE BASED ON THESE FINDINGS? Yes _____ No _____

Once I change my practice, how will I know if the change has improved the care I give?

Integrating Findings from Qualitative Studies

A somewhat tangential, but important and related, issue is how the findings of qualitative studies can be summarized. At this point there is no agreed-upon, systematic method for summing up the results of two or more qualitative research studies, and some qualitative researchers think this lack impedes the utilization of the findings from qualitative studies in clinical practice (Sandelowski, Docherty, and Emden, 1997). Several methodological approaches for integration have been tried, some involving analysis and synthesis of pooled original data and others involving aggregation of the findings, but all are in early stages of development. If two different qualitative studies provide portrayals of what it means to a person who is age 80 years or over to have open-heart surgery, and those two qualitative portrayals share some common elements but also differ in significant ways, how are we to decide which captures the reality most people experience? Beyond the obvious response that when dealing with human experience there is no such thing as one version of reality, the reviewer can consider whether differences in patients' profiles and/or settings could have resulted in two different kinds of experiences. Other times, differences in findings between two qualitative studies are less the result of diverse experiences and more the result of a different way of conceptually framing the data. Careful reading of the reports may reveal similarities in the raw data, that is, before the raw data was translated to a more conceptual level. If sufficient raw data were presented in the report, these apparent differences can often be recognized not as differences in findings but more as differences in interpretation. The issues involved in bringing the findings of qualitative research together are complex, but researchers are aware of the need to address the issue in some way and are working on several different ways of doing it (Estabrooks, Field, and Morse, 1994; Noblit and Hare, 1988; Sandelowski, Docherty, and Emden, 1977).

APPRAISING RESEARCH-BASED PRACTICE GUIDELINES

Research-based practice guidelines and protocols have been used in health care since the 1970s (Haller, Reynolds, and Horsley, 1979), but recent renewed interest in them has advanced the forms they take as well as the processes by which they are produced. Practice guidelines center on the care of a particular patient population, and "specify the processes of care that are known or believed to be associated with good outcomes" (Yoos et al., 1997, p. 51). These systematically developed guides to clinical decision making and courses of action may be formulated as formal clinical protocols put forth by a professional organization, or as a clinical path developed by a practice group to assure that they are providing the best care possible to a particular patient population. Clinical guidelines may also take the form of research-based recommendations that translate the conclusions of an M-A or integrative research review into practical action. Increasingly, research-based guidelines are part of the computerized clinical care planning, documentation, and clinical decision-making support systems used in hospitals; the research-based recommendations can be incorporated into standardized care plans, and reminders of research-based protocols can be provided.

From Evidence to Recommendations

The process by which research-based practice guidelines are developed determines whether they are credible and useful. Guidelines produced by and for a particular care giving agency have the advantage of combining research evidence with local values, resources, and perspectives. Published books of clinical pathways are available; some of these are research based, others are not. True research-based care guidelines translate the evidence from a systematic research review (previously published or conducted for the purposes of developing the guideline) into specific recommendations, decision trees, algorithms, or clinical pathways. Therefore, it is extremely important to note whether or not the process by which a guideline was produced started with a systematic summary of the research evidence bearing on each aspect of the topic the protocol addresses (Cook, Greengold, Ellrodt, and Weingarten, 1997). Because the translation from research findings to guidelines is vulnerable to bias, error, and misinterpretation, its credibility must be appraised. Beyea and Nicoll's (1995) protocol for the administration of medications via the intramuscular route is a credible guideline because it (1) is based on an extensive research review; (2) addresses each important decision point in the procedure, (3) documents the research resource for each recommended action, and (4) provides a rationale for each recommendation.

Clarity of Purpose

The information accompanying a research-based practice guideline should explicitly state what the guideline covers and does not cover and what patient group it was designed for. It should be very clear about the possible options at each decision point and about the actions recommended. The reasons why the developers recommend one option over others (or the conditions under which one option has been found to be more effective than another) should be justified. The guideline should include the outcomes associated with each course of action, and all possible outcomes of interest should be addressed (Sackett, Richardson, Rosenberg, and Haynes, 1997). In short, in the accompanying document the developers should convince you that they considered all available and relevant evidence in formulating their recommendations.

Supporting Evidence

Research-based guidelines should provide the reader at the very least with a list of the studies that support each recommendation and a discussion of the nature of the evidence. Another way of sharing the panel's evaluation of the evidence with the reader is to provide a "strength of evidence" rating for each recommendation. Several of the AHCPR clinical practice guidelines have used this approach. The panel that developed the Cardiac Rehabilitation guidelines used the strength-of-evidence ratings displayed in Box 10–1, and noted that the ratings reflect the quality of the studies on which the recommendation was based as well as the consistency of the scientific evidence (AHCPR, 1995, p. 25).

> Box 10–1
> ## AHCPR Strength of Evidence Ratings
>
> **A** = Scientific evidence provided by well-designed, well-conducted controlled trials (randomized and nonrandomized) with statistically significant results that consistently support the guideline recommendation.
>
> **B** = Scientific evidence provided by observational studies or by controlled trials with less consistent results to support the guideline recommendation.
>
> **C** = Expert opinion that supports the guideline recommendation because the available scientific evidence did not present consistent results, or controlled trials were lacking.

Current Basis

When appraising a clinical practice guideline you should take note of when the guidelines were completed as well as the latest date of the research included in the review. A clinical practice guideline should include all research conducted until just prior to the time the guideline was written. In addition, the guidelines should have been developed by panels that have a broad mix of skills and perspectives. Practitioners who will be influenced by the guideline, specialists and generalists, should participate in the development of the guidelines, as should patients who have insights into the decisions addressed by the guideline. The panel should also have at least one person who is expert in appraising research evidence. In appraising a research-based clinical practice guideline, it is fair to take into account the credentials of the members of the panel, because clinical judgments will inevitably enter into the development of clinical practice guidelines.

Comprehensiveness

The comprehensiveness of a guideline may or may not be problematic. When guideline developers limit the choice of interventions included in the guideline to a certain category of interventions—e.g., psychosocial and educational interventions for weight reduction—they are not addressing the decision in the way that the decision is experienced by practitioners and patients who will most likely have to consider the full range of interventions, e.g., special diets, diet supplements, appetite controlling medication, exercise and dietary counseling, support group involvement, and referral for anti-obesity medications or biofeedback. When confronted with a guideline that addresses only part of a decision field, you may have to supplement your decision making with other evidence.

Implementation

Recently there has been a proliferation of practice guidelines and protocols emanating from clinical specialty organizations, from government agencies, and from experts writing in professional journals. The quality of these guidelines should be appraised, and you should consider the fit between the recommendations of the guideline and the resources of your particular setting. Some guidelines are relatively easy to implement, but others are quite involved and costly. Once implemented, there should be some kind of local follow up, i.e., quality improvement evaluation, to determine if the guidelines have been correctly implemented, are being used accurately, and if improved clinical decision making and patient outcomes have been realized (Weingarten, 1997). The following questions incorporate all these aspects of appraising a clinical guideline.

Appraisal Questions

Synopsis

What does the guideline address?
What population of patients is the guideline intended for?
What are the key decision points addressed by the guideline?
What outcomes are addressed by the guideline?
What process was used to develop the guideline?

Credibility Profile

Are the guidelines based on a comprehensive meta-analysis or integrative research review?
Is the scientific basis for each recommendation provided?
Are all the key decision points addressed?
At each decision point, was the full range of actions evaluated?
Does the discussion of the way the panel reached decisions convince me that all evidence was considered in an impartial manner?
Are the guidelines current?
Was the panel that developed the guideline made up of people with the necessary skills, expertise, and backgrounds?

ARE THE RECOMMENDATIONS CREDIBLE? Yes _____ No _____

Applicability Profile

Does the guideline address a problem, decision, or situation I see in practice?
Would I be using all or just part of the guideline? Specify what parts.
Are the recommended courses of action acceptable and feasible to me and my patients?
To follow the guideline, what will I have to do differently?
Do I have the resources, skills, and equipment to implement this guideline accurately and safely?

SHOULD I ADOPT THIS GUIDELINE IN ITS ENTIRETY? Yes _____ No _____

SHOULD I ADOPT PARTS OF IT? Yes _____ No _____

What will I have to do to implement the change?
How will I know if my patients are benefiting from use of the guideline?

SUMMARY

State-of-the-science summaries of research findings, if well produced, are invaluable sources of research information for the busy practitioner, and will increasingly become essential tools for staying atop the multitude of research evidence that is being generated. However, the methods by which synthesized summaries have been produced need to be appraised to assure that the production process itself did not introduce bias, error, or oversight into the end product. Although some practitioners would like to believe that editors of clinical and research journals are screening what is published for scientific soundness, this is not a fail-safe assumption. Practitioners, as informed, responsible consumers, should be able to appraise state-of-the-science summaries for the most obvious of methodological weaknesses and to decide whether or not their findings are applicable to practice.

References

Agency for Health Care Policy and Research (1993). *Depression in Primary Care, Clinical Practice Guideline,* no. 5, vol. 2. Treatment of major depression (AHCPR publication no. 93-0551). Rockville, MD, U.S. Department of Health and Human Services.

Agency for Health Care Policy and Research (1995). *Cardiac Rehabilitation, Clinical Practice Guideline,* no. 17 (AHCPR publication no. 96-0672). U.S. Department of Health and Human Services.

Benner, P. (1984). *From Novice to Expert: Excellence and Power in Clinical Nursing Practice.* Menlo Park, CA: Addison-Wesley.

Beyea, S.C., and Nicoll, L.H. (1995). Administration of medications via the intramuscular route: An integrative review of the literature and research-based protocol for the procedure. *Applied Nursing Research,* 8:23–33.

Brown, S.A. (1991). Measurement of quality of primary studies for meta-analysis. *Nursing Research, 40,* 352–355.

Brown, S.A., and Grimes, D.E. (1993). *Nurse Practitioners and Certified Nurse-Midwives: A Meta-Analysis of Studies on Nurses in Primary Care Roles.* Washington, DC: American Nurses Publishing.

Cappelleri, J.C., Ioannidis, J.P.A., Schmid, C.H., de Ferranti, S.D., Aubert, M., Chalmers, T.C., and Lau, J. (1996). Large trials vs meta-analysis of smaller trials: How do their results compare? *Journal of American Medical Association, 276:*1332–1338.

Cook, D.J., Mulrow, C.D., and Haynes, R.B. (1997). Systematic reviews: Synthesis of best evidence for clinical decisions. *Annals of Internal Medicine, 126:*376–380.

Cook, D.J., Greengold, N.L., Ellrodt, A.G., and Weingarten, S.R. (1997). The relation between systematic reviews and practice guidelines. *Annals of Internal Medicine, 127:*210–216.

Cooper, H., and Hedges, L.V. (eds.) (1994). *The Handbook of Research Synthesis.* New York: Russell Foundation.

Cummings, P. (1994). Antibiotics to prevent infection in patients with dog bite wounds: A meta-analysis of randomized trials. *Annals of Emergency Medicine, 23*:535–540.

Devine, E.C. (1990). Meta-analysis: A new approach for reviewing research. *In* N.L. Chaska (ed.), *The Nursing Profession: Turning Points* (pp. 180–185). St. Louis: Mosby.

Dishman, R.K., and Buckworth, J. (1996). Increasing physical activity: A quantitative synthesis. *Medicine and Science in Sports and Exercise, 28*:706–719.

Eddy, D.M., and Hasselblad, V. (1994). Analyzing evidence by the confidence profile method. *In* K.A. McCormick, S.R. Moore, and R.A. Siegel (eds.), *Clinical Practice Guideline Development: Methodology Perspectives* (pp. 42–51). Agency for Health Care Policy and Research.

Estabrooks, C.A., Field, P.A., and Morse, J.M. (1994). Aggregating qualitative findings: An approach to theory development. *Qualitative Health Research, 4*:503–511.

Haller, K.B., Reynolds, M.A., and Horsley, J.A. (1979). Developing research-based innovation protocols: Process, criteria, and issues. *Research in Nursing and Health, 2*:45–51.

Laupacis, A., Sackett, D.L., and Roberts, R.S. (1988). An assessment of clinically useful measures of the consequences of treatments. *New England Journal of Medicine, 318*:1728–1733.

Massey, J., and Loomis, M. (1988). When should nurses use research findings? *Applied Nursing Research, 1*:32–40.

McCaul, K.D., Branstetter, A.D., Schroeder, B.M., and Glasgow, R.E. (1996). What is the relationship between breast cancer risk and mammography screening? A meta-analytic review. *Health Psychology, 15*:423–429.

Noblit, G.W., and Hare, R.D. (1988). *Meta-ethnography: Synthesizing Qualitative Studies.* Newbury Park, CA: Sage.

Psaty, B.M., Smith, N.L., Siscovick, D.S., Koepsell, T.D., Weiss, N.S., Heckbert, S.R., Lemaitre, R.N., Wagner, D.H., and Furberg, C.D. (1997). Health outcomes associated with antihypertensive therapies used as first-line agents: A systematic review and meta-analysis. *Journal of American Medical Association, 277*:739–745.

Reynolds, N.R., Timmerman, G., Anderson, J., and Stevenson, J.S. (1992). Meta-analysis for descriptive research. *Research in Nursing and Health, 15*:467–475.

Rosenthal, R., and Rosnow, R.L. (1984). *Essential of Behavioral Research: Methods and Data Analysis.* New York: McGraw-Hill.

Rosenthal, R. (1991). *Meta-analytic Procedures for Social Research (rev. ed.).* Newbury Park, CA: Sage.

Sackett, D.L., Richardson, W.S., Rosenberg, W., and Haynes, R.B. (1997). *Evidence-Based Medicine: How to Practice and Teach EBM.* New York: Churchill Livingstone.

Sandelowski, M., Docherty, S., and Emden, C. (1997). Qualitative metasynthesis: Issues and techniques. *Research in Nursing and Health, 20*:365–371.

Smith, K., Cook, D., Guyatt, G.H., Madhavan, J., and Oxman, A.D. (1992). Respiratory muscle training in chronic airflow limitation: A meta-analysis. *American Review of Respiratory Diseases, 145*:533–539.

Warshafsky, S., Kramer, R.S., and Sivak, S.L. (1993). Effect of garlic on total serum cholesterol: A meta-analysis. *Annals of Internal Medicine, 119*:559–605.

Weingarten, S. (1997). Editorial: Practice guidelines and prediction rules should be subject to careful clinical testing. *Journal of the American Medical Association, 277*:1977–1978.

Yoos, H.L., Malone, K., McMullen, A., Richards, K., Rideout, K., and Schultz, J. (1997). *Journal of Nursing Care Quality, 11*:48–54.

Making a Change and Evaluating Its Impact

Having reached a decision about whether you should change your practice and given some initial thought to what might be involved in making a change, you are now ready to develop a definitive plan for change and to implement it (see Figure 11–1). If you are making a change in your own practice, the situation is quite different than if you and your group are recommending a change in practice within a larger provider group. This chapter starts with a discussion of making a change in your own practice; then several points pertinent to making a research-based change in a department, agency, hospital, or health care system are presented. Finally, issues related to evaluating the effects of research-based change in individual practice and in an organization are addressed. As an additional resource, several recommended books and articles about organizational change are cited in the suggested readings in the reference list at the end of the chapter.

MAKING A CHANGE IN YOUR OWN PRACTICE

If you or your group identified the original clinical problem and traversed one of the research-based practice pathways to this point, you have examined the research evidence and made a decision to change; thus, you have personally experienced the early and middle stages of the research-based practice process. As a result, resistance to adopting that change would not seem to be an issue. Still, you may find that the actual process of moving away from routine behavior may feel like a bit of a burden. Depending on the change you are making, it may take weeks or even months before you can use the change well and without conscious effort. During the learning period required to acquire adeptness in the new approach, you may have doubts about the change. You may even be tempted to jettison the whole idea and revert to your prior way of doing things. While this reversion may

Pathways of Research-based Practice

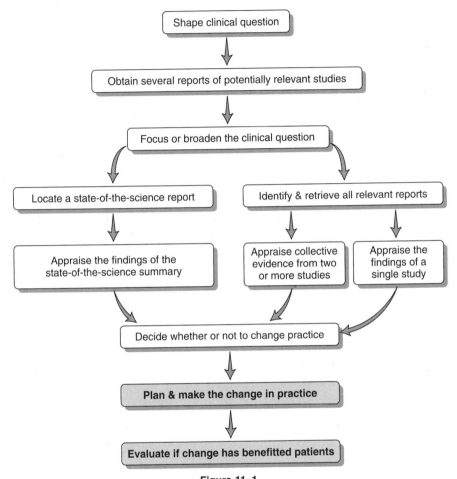

Figure 11–1.

be prudent in some situations, in many others it is merely a reaction to the awkwardness and stress of learning a new skill or behavior. If your reasons for wanting to make the change are still intact, make sure you give the change a good try by being patient and allowing yourself time to work out the glitches that weren't anticipated.

RESEARCH-BASED CHANGE IN AN ORGANIZATION

Resistance to change is more likely to be an issue when introducing an innovation that requires others to change the way they do something. Even though you (meaning you as an individual or as a group who appraised the research evidence and are recommending the change) are convinced that you are advocating a better way of doing something, you should recognize that others who have not gone through the process of appraising the research evidence as you have may not feel that the change is necessary or advantageous. Your thinking was undoubtedly changed by the process of examining the evidence, whereas they will only hear this same information second-hand, which is not as convincing as directly examining the evidence.

Persons working in almost every area of health care delivery are bombarded by new regulations, policies, equipment, forms, physical plant moves, and organizational initiatives requiring them to change how they do things. Some changes clearly produce improvement in patient care, whereas others do not. The fact that your change is based on research and has a high likelihood of improving patients' outcomes or experience of care provides a compelling rationale for it. Many people have respect for research findings—and you will want to capitalize on this fact. To do so, you should have some plan for informing them of the scientific basis for this change in an effort to influence their attitudes toward it. You may want to make one or several research abstracts or evidence reports available to people who will be affected by the change. Alternatively, you may want to include a "rationale section" in the written communication through which you announce the change—don't hesitate to briefly cite a few studies, as this can be persuasive information. Presentation of the research base will influence some persons to be receptive to the innovation, but other persons will not be swayed at all. Still, it's worth the effort as it may make some persons more aware of the fact that there is research on the topic.

One hospital had been using tympanic thermometers for approximately one year when several nurses appraised the research evidence bearing on their accuracy. They were convinced from that evidence that tympanic temperature measurements produced many false low readings and thus missed elevated temperatures. However, they thought there would be considerable resistance if they proposed going back to mercury or even electronic oral thermometers. To prepare for this resistance, they collected data comparing tympanic readings to mercury thermometer readings in two different ways. For five days they asked all care providers on a particular unit to obtain mercury thermometer readings on all patients who had a subnormal tympanic value, and on another unit they randomly (across times of day, types of patients, and care providers) obtained mercury readings in addition to tympanic readings on 100 patients. They counted the number of tympanic readings that were low by one degree or more and further analyzed the low readings and discrepancies in terms of types of patients in which they occurred. These data collection efforts established the extent to which they were getting false low readings and the extent to which they were missing elevated temperatures in their patients. Thus, instead of actually implementing a research-based change, they first collected data about how the problem identified by the research affected several populations in their setting. This local information in combination with the research on the issue provided a solid rationale for a protocol regarding the use of different kinds of thermometers in various clinical situations.

Several detailed descriptions of the implementation and evaluation of research-based practice innovations have been compiled in one volume of *The Nursing Clinics of North America* (Titler and Goode, 1995). The examples include latex allergy precautions, dressings for peripheral intravenous catheter sites, and animal-assisted therapy in a critical care setting; a wide variety of outcomes data and other quality information were used in the evaluations.

EVALUATING THE CHANGE IN INDIVIDUAL OR SMALL GROUP PRACTICE

Generally, the amount of effort put into evaluating effects of a change should be somewhat in proportion to the potential risks and benefits to patients as well as to the resources expended to implement the change. You want to obtain reliable and meaningful information, but you don't want the evaluation process to become a burden. In planning an evaluation of the effects of a research-based change, you need to keep in mind that your purpose is evaluation, not the conduct of research.

Data Sources and Data Management

Data Logs

In an office setting your evaluation effort could consist of a log where you systematically record the names of the patients with whom you used the change and any information that you need to reach a conclusion regarding the effectiveness of the intervention or approach. It is highly advantageous if this log can be set up or the data transferred to a spread sheet, as this will greatly ease and enhance the analysis of data. It's best if you give some advance thought to what information you need rather than just making a narrative entry; consider setting up the log in columns for quick, concise entries. The most important forms of information will be clinical indicators reflecting the patients' status at each visit such as physical findings, vital signs, or laboratory values, and patients' reports of how they have been feeling or what they have been experiencing in their daily lives. You will get some ideas regarding what clinical indicators and patients' reports to record from the dependent variables used in the studies you have appraised. Once you have 10 to 20 entries in your log, you can begin to look for patterns indicating improved outcomes, no change in outcomes, or adverse consequences of having made the change. You will probably find it useful to tally your data in the form of percentage of patients falling into each outcome category, but you should also look for any recurring data suggestive of unanticipated benefits or problems. Regardless of how you analyze your log data, the systematic process of your evaluation effort will undoubtedly yield valuable information and insights regarding the effects of your research-based practice in particular but also about your patients more generally.

Chart Audits

Rather than keep a data log you may prefer to keep a list of persons who have received, used, or been exposed to the new approach. Once you have a reasonable number, retrieve those charts and extract the data you need to evaluate how well the innovation is working. Your audit will be more worthwhile if you give some thought to what information you want to document in your clinical notes so the audit results will be more meaningful and complete. Using a preplanned data recording form will enable you to extract the information quickly and objectively, and it will be easier to analyze; this is particularly true if the data form uses yes-no questions, simple counts, and predetermined categories.

Information from Patients

Most evaluation of research-based change should include a focus on patients' perceptions of how the change has affected them. Too often providers decide what the meaningful outcomes should be and ask patients about them, rather than first providing opportunity for patients to express what they view as good, bad, and inconsequential about a new therapy or approach. Not infrequently, patients identify different outcomes and issues than providers identify. For example, in eliciting patients' perceptions of outcomes associated with a complimentary therapy, several patients mentioned feeling more calm, in control, and clear-thinking after the therapy, whereas providers wanted to ask them about the effects the therapy had on disease- and treatment-related symptoms such as nausea, pain, and shortness of breath. The important point of this as it relates to evaluating a research-based change is to first give patients an opportunity to express what they value and how they see things without imposing issues, and only after they have expressed their views should the person eliciting the data ask specific questions (May, 1991). This guideline applies equally to one-on-one interviews and to focus group interviewing.

When asking patients at a visit to estimate the frequency of an experience in daily life, the best approach is probably to ask them what their experience has been during the last week, because that's about all you can expect people to remember accurately. For experiences that occur at infrequent or irregular intervals, you may get more accurate information if you ask the patient to keep a diary or log at home and make an entry every day. The frequency and time period for keeping such a diary should be as short as possible to avoid imposing a burden on patients that will result in low levels of completion.

You may want to go beyond informal questions and ask the patients to complete a questionnaire that was developed specifically for the evaluation or that was used in one of the studies. If this is done, you obviously need to provide some explanation regarding what is being asked and plan time and space for them to complete the written materials. Because you are evaluating a change, not doing research, you don't have to use the entire questionnaire as it was developed and used in the research study. You can extract sections or just those questions that pertain to the change you have made; alternatively, you can make a composite of questions from several instruments that serves your purposes better than any existing one does. It is important that the format be clear and easy for patients to complete, which may require that you pilot test it on three to five patients.

Focus Groups

Another approach to evaluation that incorporates patients' perspectives is the use of focus groups (Beaudin and Pelletier, 1996; Patton, 1990). Within the context of evaluation of a clinical service, a focus group is a group interview by which four to eight persons who have received the new service or therapy provide information and feedback regarding their experiences of that care and its effectiveness. The care being evaluated can be the totality of care received or some particular aspect of it.

Focus groups work best when the interviewer sets forth the purpose of the interview, has prepared four to eight clear questions, and has skill in facilitating group discussion. Typically focus groups with a purpose of evaluating a new clinical service last 30 to 60 minutes, and are audiotaped for subsequent analysis. The first three or four questions should be broad and open-ended, which will allow the participants' views of the care to be elicited and are intended to encourage all persons to contribute. When not all persons who received the service will be asked to participate in the focus groups, some type of random or stratified sampling should be used to invite participants so as to avoid bias in who contributes information to the evaluation.

Short Interviews

You should also give thought to what persons other than patients might have an important perspective on whether the change has made a difference and try to obtain information from them. Such persons could include patients' families, a specialty provider to whom you refer patients, or a school nurse. Sometimes, a short face-to-face or telephone interview consisting of five or six questions will provide very useful information with the least amount of work. It can be informal, but the information obtained should be written up for subsequent analysis; often a secretarial person can be trained to make the contact, ask the questions, and record the answers.

Physiologic Data

Often physiologic data collected in the course of providing care can be used to evaluate whether a change in practice is producing the anticipated benefit. Physiologic monitoring values such as oxygen saturation levels and intercranial pressures are frequently determined and recorded as part of the routine clinical management of certain patient populations. Routinely obtained laboratory values can serve also as indicators of the success of a new approach to care. For example, urine cultures can be used to determine whether an approach to preventing urinary tract infections is effective, and the glycosylated hemoglobin test can be used as an indicator of diabetic self-management over a 6- to 12-week period.

Other physiologic data are not routinely recorded and special plans must be made for collecting them; for example, sleep-awake periods are not routinely recorded, nor are patients' levels of agitation quantified using a scale, nor are the frequency, intensity, and location of post-stroke patients' muscle spasms in the affected side muscles systematically recorded in most settings. When the desired data are not routinely recorded, it is usually advantageous to use a structured approach to recording the data, such as definitions to go with the descriptive terms the recorder will be using. Alternatively, a numerical scale could be used to quantify observations of a particular patient state and care providers trained in its use.

Concurrent, or real time, recording of the desired data can be done in ways that ensure that there is consistency in the use of scales, values, terms, and units. However, care must be taken when asking clinicians to make special determinations and recordings, lest patient care be compromised by adding to the providers' workload. Retrospective extraction of the data from patients' records avoids this burden, but record data is typically incomplete or inconsistently recorded.

Analysis of Evaluation Data

Evaluation of a new approach or therapy inevitably raises the issue of "What criteria do I use to decide that the change has had a meaningful impact?" The answer depends on the nature of the change and on how involved you want to get in the evaluation process. The best way, of course, would be to have baseline data taken before the change on these patients to compare the post-change data to, but that may not be possible for a variety of reasons. Alternatively, you may have pre-change data on a similar group of patients who received either no treatment or a different treatment, and this data can serve as a baseline for deciding whether patients receiving the new treatment are experiencing better outcomes. In either case you should determine in advance a level of improvement that you expect; this level could be determined by what levels of outcomes were found in the research, by what constitutes an improvement over your previous level of outcomes, or by some combination of these two considerations.

The following example illustrates the evaluation options just described. Suppose the staff of a pain clinic wanted to evaluate a new reserach-based approach they were using for a certain population of patients. They could ask patients to keep track of when their pain experiences interfered with their daily lives in important ways. Patients could be asked to write on a special calendar when they were not able to go to work or school, when they were not able to fulfill their family or household responsibilities, and when they were not able to participate in a social or recreational activity in which they would have liked to be involved.

The program could be considered a success if each of these interferences with daily life was reduced by 20 percent in 80 percent of the people in the group (assuming that this target represents a clinically meaningful effect). However, this approach would require obtaining baseline data before instituting the new approach, something that may not be possible to do. Alternatively, if research data regarding the effects of similar approaches on social functioning were available, the clinic staff might know that a target level of less than two job-school interferences and less than 10 responsibility-social-recreational interferences per month in 85 percent of the people is indicative of program success. The advantage of basing the target on outcome data from research is that it would require only a post-intervention data collection to determine if the program were achieving good outcomes. Clearly, target setting requires clinical understanding of what outcomes and outcome levels are desirable and creativity to identify outcome-related data that is feasible to obtain, as well as knowledge about the research base on the clinical topic.

There will be situations in which you do not have access to baseline data of any sort, in which case you would just maintain your log or keep a list of patients receiving the new treatment so you can perform a chart audit once enough people have received the new therapy or treatment approach. Your conclusions would be based on the treated group alone, not on any comparison. Here, again, you need to remember that you are not conducting research. To reach a conclusion about the effectiveness of the change in your practice, you just need to systematically and objectively summarize whatever data you have and compare that to a target level of outcome achievement that you view as clinically meaningful. Your target level may even need to be based on a rough "guesstimate" of what outcome levels you were achieving prior to making the research-based change.

ORGANIZATIONAL APPROACHES TO EVALUATING RESEARCH-BASED CHANGE

When evaluating the effects of research-based changes within a larger health care organization or system, your evaluation plan may be more ambitious, because more extensive data sources and retrieval capability are often available. Many of the tools and data systems used by your quality improvement programs to monitor and evaluate service product lines will be useful in evaluating the impact of a research-based innovation. Evaluation data can be obtained using the following:

- Patient surveys,
- Reviews/audits of patients' records for key process and outcomes indicators,
- Extraction of relevant indicators from existing administrative databases,
- Data collection tools developed by the organization, and
- Special arrangements for obtaining data from other providers or other databases.

Impact on Outcomes

By examining the outcomes and the ways in which the outcomes were measured in the research studies, those planning an evaluation of a research-based innovation may obtain useful ideas about what kinds of evaluation data would be meaningful. It is critical to identify the outcomes that should be realized if the research-based change is having its intended effect, and what indicators could be used to determine whether those outcomes have been achieved or not. Then a specific plan for collecting data regarding those indicators should be developed. It may also be advisable to consider what adverse outcomes might occur as a result of the innovation and collect data regarding their occurrence. The number of outcome indicators in the evaluation plan should be feasible to obtain and analyze, given the systems and resources of the organization.

Patient Outcomes

Certainly, patient outcomes should have a central place in the evaluation of a research-based innovation in an organization, just as they do in individual and small group practice. Beyond the types of information that can be obtained directly from patients and their health care records, large organizations often have sources of data regarding population outcomes that are not available to individual and small practices. Data regarding utilization patterns within a health care system and profiles of patient populations may be useful in evaluating the effects of an innovation; aggregate data such as number and types of services used, in-hospital complication rates, co-morbidity patterns, referral patterns, procedure rates, and total charges are often attainable from the organization's administrative databases. Also, it may be possible to obtain aggregate data from other sources such as the databases of insurers, HMOs, states, municipalities, and special clinical registries. Special arrangements for obtaining individual data from other agencies or health care providers can also be useful (e.g., days missed from school, frequency of participation in facility social events, return to work rates). Large organizations often have the resources to develop special tools to evaluate the effects of care within their setting (e.g., questionnaires, rating scales, performance tests). Alternatively, a research measurement tool could be adapted to the organization's unique concerns and values.

Summing up the Data

Analysis of outcome data need not involve inferential statistics, although it may. Generally, descriptive statistics such as averages, ranges, counts, percentages, and percentiles provide sufficient information to decide if an innovation is having a positive effect. In a research utilization project aimed at decreasing patient falls in a hospital, the effectiveness of a research-based fall prevention program was evaluated by comparing the rate of falls before the intervention to that after the intervention (Kilpack, Boehm, Smith, and Mudge, 1991). This was done by counting the number of falls in the year prior to the program and the number in the year following the program, and by calculating the fall rate per 1000 patient days (fall rate = number of falls/number of patient days $\times$ 1000), which is a useful way of giving standardized meaning to the number of falls. Also important was the fact that they analyzed fall rates in light of changes in patient acuity and staffing. This report illustrates how easily calculated numbers can convey a clear sense of a program's effect on patient outcomes, and how other factors in the situation that may have influenced the outcomes can be taken into account.

Evaluation, Not Research

Because the task at hand is evaluation of how an innovation is working in a specific setting, not research, the data collection plan should be objective, feasible, and meaningful to those in the setting; research methods such as control of individual differences, use of a control group, and random assignment to a treatment group are not necessary. However, random sampling is a valuable tool in evaluation, just as it is in conducting research. Its use reduces the amount of data that needs to be collected to ensure that the data obtained is representative of the population's data. Some organizations may be able to mount evaluation projects that methodologically approach research standards, whereas other organizations will have to be more modest in their evaluation of research-based change. Regardless of scale and rigor, the evaluation effort should provide objective and reliable information regarding whether the patients who received or were exposed to the innovation in your organization are achieving expected outcomes at levels that were anticipated.

Feedback to Providers

Once evaluative data has been obtained, it is particularly important that the information be looped back in a timely way to the providers who have been part of the change. This feedback may be in the form of information about the outcomes an individual practitioner's patients are achieving or in the more general form of the outcomes the patient population is achieving. If the change has been difficult for practitioners to adopt, early quality improvement data showing improved patient outcomes may bolster them in their adjustment to the new approach. Even if the change was easy to implement, hearing that it has changed patient outcomes or satisfaction is usually welcome reinforcement, and may pave the road for future research-based changes. And if no improvement has been realized, this needs to be taken into account and the approach either fine-tuned, given more emphasis with the staff, or abandoned.

One nursing department, after having made a research-based change in protocols aimed at preventing and reducing falls, had five nurses from each unit audit the charts of patients who had fallen while on their unit to determine if the protocols had been followed and whether the falls might have been prevented. Once ten patient falls had occurred on the unit, an audit group was mobilized which produced a report that was posted on the unit within days and then discussed at the next staff meeting. The short time frame between the fall occurrences and when the staff was given information about patterns in the occurrence of the falls and opportunity to plan corrective action constituted a quick response assuring that the research-based protocols were being followed. Although the main purpose of the chart review was to determine if and how the new protocols were not being followed, additional benefits were realized as the nurses who conducted the reviews became more aware of the many factors that contribute to patient falls. This chart review worked in combination with their usual continuous quality improvement reports about patient falls on their units to provide considerable information about the extent to which the research-based change in the processes of care was influencing patient outcomes.

SUMMARY

Only when evaluation of a research-based change has been completed has a practitioner or practice group traversed the entire length of a research-based pathway. Some practitioners find the evaluation stage a rewarding part of the journey, whereas others find it superfluous as they feel they already know if the change has benefited patients or not. The reality is, however, that systematic evaluation is necessary to assure objectivity and to generate supporting data for those who might need to justify the cost of the change to third-party payers or budgetary overseers.

Evaluation of the change completes the research-based practice journey by linking the activities undertaken back to the original purpose of obtaining research-based evidence to answer a specific clinical question in a particular setting. By seeking research-based answers to clinical questions, practitioners enact their commitment to providing patients with the best care possible— care that incorporates all the sources of evidence available to contemporary providers.

References

Beaudin C.L., and Pelletier, L.R. (1996). Consumer-based research: Using focus groups as a method for evaluating quality of care. *Journal of Nursing Care Quality,* *10*:28–33.

Kilpack, V., Boehm, J., Smith, N., and Mudge, B. (1991). Using research-based interventions to decrease patient falls. *Applied Nursing Research,* *4*(2):50–56.

May, K.A. (1991). Interview techniques in qualitative research: Concerns and challenges. *In* Morse, J.M. (ed.). *Qualitative Nursing Research: A Contemporary Dialogue.* Newbury Park, CA: Sage (pp. 188–201).

Patton, M.Q. (1990). *Qualitative Evaluation and Research Methods,* 2*nd* ed. Newbury Park, CA: Sage.

Titler, M.G., and Goode, C.J. (eds.) (1995). Research utilization. *The Nursing Clinics of North America,* *30*(3).

Suggested Readings Regarding Organizational Change

Barnsteiner, J.H. (1996). Research-based practice. *Nursing Administration Quarterly,* *20*(4):52–58.

Brill, P.L., and Worth, R. (1997). *The Four Levers of Corporate Change.* New York: Amacon.

Bostrom, J., and Wise, L. (1994). Closing the gap between research and practice. *Journal of Nursing Administration,* *24*(5):22–27.

Champagne, M.T., Tornquist, E.M., and Funk, S.G. (1997). Achieving research-based practice. *American Journal of Nursing,* *97*(5):16AAA–16DDD.

Cronenwett, L.R. (1992). Using research in practice. *In* Funk, S.G., et al. (eds.) (1992). *Key Aspects of Elder Care: Falls, Incontinence, and Cognitive Impairment.* New York: Springer (pp. 28–38).

Horsley, J., Crane, J., Crabtree, M., and Wood, D. (1983). *Using Research to Improve Nursing Practice: A Guide.* New York: Grune & Stratton.

Kitson, A., Ahmed, L.B., Harvey, G., Seers, K., and Thompson, D.R. (1996). From research to practice: one organizational model for promoting research-based practice. *Journal of Advanced Nursing, 23*:430–440.

LaMarsh, J. (1995). *Changing the Way We Change: Gaining Control of Major Organizational Change.* Reading, MA: Addison-Wesley.

Larsen, L.L., and Thurston, N.E. (1997). Research utilization: development of central venous catheter procedure. *Applied Nursing Research, 10*:44–51.

Meyer, A.D., and Goes, J.B. (1988). Organizational assimilation of innovation: A multilevel contextual analysis. *Academy of Management Journal, 3*:897–923.

Niesen, K.M., and Quirk, A.G. (1997). The process for initiating nursing practice changes in the intrapartum: findings from a multisite research utilization project. *Journal of Obstetric, Gynecologic, and Neonatal Nursing, 26*:709–717.

Rutledge, D.N., Greene, P., Mooney, K., Nail, L.M., and Ropka, M. (1996). Use of research-based practices by oncology staff nurses. *Oncology Nursing Forum, 23*:1235–1244.

VandenBosch, T.M., Cooch, J., and Treston-Aurand, J. (1997). Research utilization: adhesive bandage dressing regimen for peripheral venous catheters. *American Journal of Infection Control, 25*:513–519.

Williams, K.S., Crichton, N.J., and Roe, B. (1997). Disseminating research evidence: A controlled trial in continence care. *Journal of Advanced Nursing, 25*:691–698.

Committing to Research-Based Practice

The integration of research findings into professional health care practice is currently receiving considerable attention, but in reality it has always been part of professional health care practice. What is new about the heightened interest in the utilization of research findings is the recognition that it is indeed a complex activity. The informed consumer of health care research needs to have sufficient knowledge of how research should be done in order to (a) sort through published studies and decide which findings are credible and which are not; (b) see patterns, inconsistencies, and contradictions in findings from several studies on the same topic; and (c) decide whether a summary of evidence compiled by someone else is credible. Considering the large number of studies being conducted, the wide variety of research designs in use, and the increasing number of research summaries being published, knowledge required to perform these basic research utilization activities is extensive. In addition, when deciding whether and how to transfer research findings into practice, practitioners often have to translate findings into clinically meaningful terms because researchers don't consistently provide useful clinical interpretations of their findings. Thus, substantial knowledge of research methodology is required to appraise the credibility and clinical significance of findings and collective evidence.

ACKNOWLEDGING THE COMPLEXITY

In acknowledgment of this complexity, the evidence-based practice movement has tackled the difficult task of detailing the specific aspects of study design that must be considered when appraising research findings. The specification has focused largely on the appraisal of findings from single studies, but has also spelled out the issues that affect the credibility of meta-analysis. This book has been an attempt to fill in some of the ground that the evidence-based practice movement, which has been most active in medicine, has not addressed. This neglected ground includes (a) the appraisal of findings from qualitative, descriptive, and correlational studies; (b) the appraisal of collective evidence from two or more studies;

(c) and evidence from integrative research reviews and research-based clinical protocols.

At present members of the health care disciplines are on the upward slope of a learning curve where we are learning to be both skeptical and open to research finding and to appreciate the contributions of a wide variety of study designs. We are learning new strategies for combining evidence from across several studies and how to decide if findings and research evidence are likely to hold up in our setting. And we are learning how to weave research findings and evidence together with the other sources of evidence that influence clinical decision making.

In the past there was an expectation that health care providers would use research findings in their practice, but there was little specific guidance regarding how to appraise a collective body of findings about a topic or how to appraise the readiness of findings for practice. The current research-based practice movement, or evidence-based practice movement, offers detailed guidance in the form of specific appraisal questions for various types of evidence. As you can tell from the questions provided in this book, the questions that have been developed approach appraisal from the perspective of practice, not from the perspective of methodological critique. Moreover, the questions probe the credibility, clinical significance, and applicability of findings deeply. Admittedly, the knowledge and critical thinking skills required to engage in research-based practice as it has been presented in this book are considerable, but they are attainable. And once acquired, they provide access to a whole new way of thinking about practice.

Some health care disciplines are further down the road in using research-based knowledge than others. More research has been done in the issues of interest to some health care disciplines than in those of interest to others—there are many historical, political, and social reasons why this is so. Research into diseases and disease treatment clearly has been funded to a much greater extent than research about how persons, couples, and families deal with life-threatening diagnoses or live with chronic illnesses. However, the human response issues are beginning to receive more research attention and funding, as are health and health care issues such as prevention, complimentary therapies, quality of life, and functioning in daily life. The reality is that research findings relevant to the full breadth of health care practice are becoming increasingly available.

COMMITMENTS AT SEVERAL LEVELS

Individual

Research-based practice is enacted at the individual, practice group, and organizational or agency level; hence, if research-based practice is to become part of the culture of practice, there must be commitment at all levels. To employ research-based practice in the way it has been presented in this book requires that you as an individual be reflective and inquisitive—reflective enough to recognize situations in your practice that you are not handling in the best way possible because you lack current and complete knowledge; inquisitive enough to want research evidence to answer your clinical questions and dilemmas and to expend effort in pursuit of that evidence.

Individuals must also be committed to developing the skills required to search databases for relevant studies, read reports and research summaries critically, and appraise findings and collective evidence. You, as the reader of this book, having reached this last chapter, have clearly made the initial commitment required to acquire these skills; however, the skills will develop more fully over time as you engage in the activities within each pathway and through dialogue with colleagues. At times this ongoing learning will be intriguing and rewarding; at other times, it may be experienced as a burden, another activity making a demand on your time.

Practitioners with a commitment to acquiring and using research-based knowledge will seek out clinical continuing education programs that incorporate research on the clinical issues being addressed into the content of the program. If a continuing education program does not include the research-based rationale for the recommendations made during the program, practitioners should ask for it either in the dialogue of the session or on the evaluation form. In this scientific era, health care practitioners should expect and demand continuing education content that is research-based to the greatest extent feasible for the subject matter of the program.

Managing Information

A major difficulty in basing practice on research evidence is that all health care practitioners are faced with an overwhelming amount of information that they must manage in order to provide high-quality health care. Research evidence is only one category of information that must be managed.[1] An important part of managing information is sorting through what presents itself and eliminating what is not relevant. However, even what seems relevant must then be appraised for credibility—one simply cannot accept information without assessing its authenticity and credibility. Fortunately, this problem is being addressed in the form of an increase in the number of state-of-the-science summaries and evidence reports from respected sources. In the near future, practitioners will undoubtedly come to rely even more on

---

[1]Among the others are new product and technology information; the rules, codes, and requirements of several reimbursement systems; risk management and liability advice; proposed and actual changes in state practice regulations regarding professional practice; financial information about the status of the practice or department; and patterns of practice and outcomes information produced by insurers and managed-care organizations.

these summative forms of research evidence; therefore, acquiring skill in appraising them will become increasingly important.

Sharing Research Evidence with Patients

Another important skill that will be required of individual practitioners is sharing research findings and research evidence with patients and their families as part of decision making regarding care, treatment, and management. Skill will be required to discern how to present the information to patients in ways that don't overwhelm them with too much detail or leave them feeling that you are giving them the information so they can make the decision by themselves. The research information must be shared in ways that invite patients to participate in decisions with you, and don't leave them feeling that you are abdicating decision-making responsibility. Presenting research evidence to patients will require some forethought about how to convey the research evidence in lay language. Your presentation should impart (1) whether there is a great deal of evidence in support of a certain approach, no evidence, or mixed findings, (2) what benefits are likely to be realized and which ones are more in doubt, and (3) separate likely adverse outcomes from uncommon ones. You need not feel obligated to present findings and evidence independent of your appraisal of them; you should feel free to express your views regarding the meaning of findings, particularly as they apply to the patient with whom you are talking.

The public is increasingly well informed about recent research, but will require help in sorting through what is applicable to a given situation, what is media hype from what is substantial and credible evidence, and what the research findings really mean. A few patients will want to read a state-of-the-science report on an issue relevant to their condition if it is offered. For instance, a well-educated or well-read 50 year old professional man with prostate cancer might want to read a state-of-the-science summary regarding the effects of hormonal regimens when used in combination with radiation therapy or surgery in the management of locally advanced prostatic cancer (Eulau and Corn, 1996). Such an article would be technically difficult but not impossible to read, and certain individuals will want to see the evidence for themselves. There is no reason why they shouldn't, particularly if the report has been chosen because it is applicable to their situation. Better that they be directed to a state-of-the-science summary that applies to their situation than having them seek out one on their own that may not be applicable.

Other issues for which some patients might appreciate being able to read a state-of-the-science summary are: comparison of the success of exercise, medical, and surgical management of back pain; prevention and management of urinary tract infections; timing of childhood immunizations; and risk versus benefit of mammography for a specific age group. Other patients will not have a need to read the evidence themselves, but will still appreciate knowing that research has been done on the therapy or approach, and that their provider is taking this into account when making a recommendation.

Practice Groups

The practice group may be the most important level of professional interaction for promoting research-based practice, because it is at this level that substantive issues can be discussed. It is at this level that individuals can be interpersonally bolstered in their research-based practice endeavors by others, and it is at this level that research knowledge can be brought to bear on the care of specific patient populations. Members of a practice group often have daily contact with one another and opportunity to discuss dilemmas in care while these issues are still prominent and fresh in their thoughts. In addition, they often see some of the same patients or the same kinds of patients, which can produce a commonality that makes the introduction of research findings into the conversation a collegial happening, rather than a scholarly pretense.

In some health care practices, reference to recent research findings regularly enters professional dialogue. A copy of a relevant study is circulated to members of the practice team; each practitioner is in touch with the research being produced relevant to the areas managed and feels responsible for bringing this to the others' attention; or individual members of the practice make a point of keeping current regarding the research on a particular topic and become known as the person to talk with to learn about the latest research on that topic. These are signs that research-based knowledge is integrally woven into the health care practice culture. In other practice groups this may not be the case. Discussion of research findings does not regularly enter into discussion of how to manage a particular case or the problems experienced by a population of patients; members of the group do not take pride in being current about research and being aware of how experts view that research. A practice group in which discussion of current research knowledge is regularly part of clinical discussions is likely to be a practice group with good clinical outcomes because the research findings constantly challenge them to think about whether current practice is effective—and that challenge keeps clinical thinking nimble and sensitive.

Health Care Systems and Organizations

Health care systems and organizations demonstrate a commitment to research-based practice by providing time for individual practitioners to locate, read, and appraise research reports. For an organization to say, "We are committed to evidence-based practice," but not provide time for all professional practitioners to locate, read, appraise, and even discuss research evidence is hypocrisy. The greatest organizational barriers to the use of research findings as perceived by American nurses in two large surveys were lack of time to implement new ideas and to read research, lack of authority to change patient care procedures, and lack of support and cooperation from others in the setting (Funk, Champagne, Tornquist, et al., 1995; Pettengill, Gillies, and Clark, 1994). If time is not provided for locating, reading, and appraising research findings, professional providers are placed in the position of knowing that relevant research evidence is available but not being able to use it to improve care because of the direct patient care load imposed by the system for which they work.

At the organizational level, no clinical pathway or new clinical program, should be developed without examining the research on the topic. In addition, standards committees and continuous quality improvement projects should be committed to bringing research findings to their deliberations and products. The use of research findings in practice should be part of every professional provider's job description—research-based practice should be expected and role incumbents should be held accountable for the activities required to enact it.

The leaders of an organization, of course, have the reciprocal responsibility for creating the conditions and providing the resources requisite to enacting research-based practice. Database searching hardware and software should be readily accessible; library resources to assist in searching for and obtaining research reports should be provided; and time for reading and appraising research evidence should be allocated in every professional's work schedule. In addition, whenever a new patient care product is proposed there should be an expectation that research evidence regarding the effectiveness of that product will be presented as part of the proposal.

Research Evidence and Quality Improvement Data

Research evidence and quality information data both contribute evidence to contemporary health care, but the relationship between these two forms of evidence is not as clear as it needs to be (Cronenwett, 1997). Research and quality improvement activities produce unique forms of knowledge; thus, a distinction between them is possible. Research produces explanatory knowledge regarding health care methods, processes, experiences, and events. Research also establishes assuredness regarding the cause-and-effect relationships between therapies, treatments, provider actions, and patient outcomes. In contrast, quality improvement activities provide practical data pertaining to the degree to which desirable outcomes are being achieved by certain patient populations over time (Lynn, 1996). Quality improvement projects are also interested in establishing linkage between processes of care and patient outcomes, hence data about whether critical process events are occurring in a timely manner are frequently obtained and analyzed.

The goal of research is to produce general knowledge that explains how the empirical world works across a broad range of situations. The goal of quality improvement information, on the other hand, is to improve the health care methods used in a specific organization or benchmarking network. In a sense, then, both knowledge endeavors have as a goal improving the care patients receive, but contribute a different form of knowledge to that improvement.

The two endeavors should augment and fuel each other. The general knowledge produced by research is put into use by practitioners in particular settings. Once the knowledge has been in use a while, there should be a check on whether it is producing the benefits that were anticipated. Information obtained in checking on the effectiveness of the knowledge when applied in real-world circumstances often reveals inconsistencies, variations, and issues that were not taken into consideration in the research that produced the general knowledge; thus, the evaluation endeavor forces refinement of the general knowledge claim. Unfortunately, the nature of this circuitous relationship has not yet been fully examined in today's health care literature. As a result, the synergy between research evidence and quality improvement data in improving health care practice has not been fully realized.

The challenges facing clinical and administrative leaders in health care organizations involve learning when to use research methods, when to use quality improvement methods, when a hybrid method with features of each knowledge producing method should be used, and how to bring the two knowledge producing tools into relationship with one another. The exploration of their relationship is beyond the scope of this book, but the author is convinced that the distinction between them serves a purpose and that further work needs to be done to explore how the two forms of knowledge augment and advance each other.

Research Evidence and Continuing Education

Organizations and educational institutions that provide professional continuing education should commit to requiring speakers to address the research that has and is being done on the topic. Speakers at continuing educational programs should be explicit in recognizing the type of evidence on which they base their recommendations; too often this is fuzzy and the attending learner cannot discern the basis for various claims made by the speakers. Research findings should be part of *every* continuing education program; they should be integrally woven into the content presented; the strength of the research evidence should be described; and study citations should be made available to attendees.

In summary, when research-based practice is genuinely adopted as an organization value, it should infuse all the activities of the organization. It should become an essential element in the atmosphere of the setting; it should become part of the language and thinking of the organization. Clinical leaders in all health care disciplines should transmit research-based practice as both a value and an expectation, and should lead by making it an integral part of everyday discourse. Administrative leaders should also commit to research-based practicing by seeking and using research evidence in health care planning, and by creating a work environment in which research-based practice is fostered.

Colleges, Universities, and Professional Schools

Finally, research-based practice should be advanced as a value in professional health care education. Research findings should be an integral part of all content and of most classroom dialogue regarding clinical care. Early in a program, not late, professional health care students should be taught how to locate and appraise research findings. They are not complex skills that should be reserved until the end of the program; instead, they are fundamental skills that should be taught early so the student has opportunity to practice them throughout the program. They are essential to learning to read the clinical literature of every professional health care discipline.

Statistics and research courses should emphasize developing the knowledge to read and appraise research, not to conduct research, and the texts used should assume the perspective and language of being an informed consumer of research knowledge. In addition, when choosing clinical texts the extent to which research-based knowledge is included and study citations provided should be considered. In short, during professional education the high value the discipline places on being an informed consumer of research-based knowledge should be conveyed explicitly, early, and consistently.

CONCLUSION: A POSSIBLE FUTURE

In the near future we may all come to rely on certified "evidence experts"—these people would specialize in the appraisal and synthesis of research evidence. In an informal sense these people already exist as those professional providers we recognize as having special skills in synthesizing results from several or many studies and in appraising research evidence across studies. The evidence experts should, of course, always work in close cooperation with researchers and practitioners in the field as research evidence is best appraised within the contexts of what is already known and not yet known, as well as what constitutes routine and feasible practice.

If cooperative endeavors between evidence experts, practitioners, and researchers, which we could call research evidence teams, come into broad existence, practitioners would be truly supported in their efforts to base practice on research evidence. Practitioners could then devote less attention to appraising the credibility and clinical significance of research evidence and devote more attention to judging the applicability of the summary knowledge to their settings and evaluating the benefits realized from making research-based changes in practice. This narrower focus would require less time than when, as now, they must also appraise the credibility of findings from individual studies and the meaning of a collective body of evidence. In addition, this shift and narrowing of focus would enable the special perspective of practitioners to be brought to bear on the issues for which they have the greatest expertise, and in many cases the greatest interest. For now and the immediate future, however, practitioners in all the health care disciplines must be able to comfortably use all the pathways of research-based practice in their entirety if they are to provide health care that is based on credible, current scientific knowledge.

References

Cronenwett, L. (1997, April). *Using Research Data in Clinical Practice: New Questions, Models, and Methods.* Paper presented at the University of North Carolina–Chapel Hill School of Nursing, the 1997 Kemble Lecture.

Eulau, S.M., and Corn, B.W. (1996). Combinations of hormones and local therapies in locally advanced prostate carcinoma. *Oncology, 10:*1193–1202.

Funk, S.G., Champagne, M.T., Tornquist, E.M., et al. (1995). Barriers to using research findings in practice: The clinician's perspective. *Applied Nursing Research, 4:*90–95.

Long, A.F., and Dixon, P. (1996). Monitoring outcomes in routine practice: Defining appropriate measurement criteria. *Journal of Evaluation in Clinical Practice, 2:*71–78.

Lynn, P.A. (1996). Relationship between total quality management, critical paths, and outcomes management. *Seminars for Nurse Managers, 4:*163–167.

Pettengill, M.M., Gillies, D.A., Clark, C.C. (1994). Factors encouraging and discouraging the use of nursing research findings. *IMAGE: Journal of Nursing Scholarship, 26:*144–147.

Appendix A. **Manual Searching**

Manual searching involves looking through bound volumes of indexes and other directories, which are organized by year, topic, or author name, to locate relevant references. The indexed references may be journal articles, books, or studies. Many printed indexes and catalogs are being moved into computerized files and in many cases are no longer available in printed form.

JOURNAL ARTICLE INDEXES

The principal index of the health sciences journal literature is Index Medicus, which has been printed since 1879. For comprehensively searching the nursing literature, the Cumulative Index to Nursing and Allied Health Literature (CINAHL) offers indexing back to the later 1950s. Both indexes offer author and subject approaches *by year* and provide authors, article title, journal title and volume, number and pages. Note that you must search each year separately. Clinical topics or questions which include more than one topic must be looked up separately under each subject. The names of multiple authors should also be looked up separately in order to assure a complete list, because indexing depends on who is the first, or primary, author of an article. The journal literature of Index Medicus prior to 1966 and of CINAHL prior to 1982 is accessible only via manual searching.

Another method for looking for journal articles is to review an index of a particular journal, many of which publish annual or semiannual indexes by author, article title, or topic. This, of course, will only get you to the articles published in one journal, and several journal indexes would have to be searched to obtain a comprehensive view of the topic.

A list of journal titles is published annually in *Ulrich's International Directory.* The directory can be searched via specific journal title or by discipline, and is useful when you want to know all the journals published in a particular field.

BOOK CATALOGS

Searching for books on a particular topic may be undertaken in several different ways. Libraries use card catalogs (most are now on computer files) to list the books owned in that particular library, so sources found in this way would not be comprehensive. Searching in *Books in Print* would add to the comprehensiveness, but still would not access books that are out of print and subject searching would be challenging. Specific libraries such as the National Library of Medicine or the library of a clinical specialty organization may be sources to contact for additional comprehensiveness in searching for relevant books.

SUMMARY

Manual searching has the advantage of not requiring a computer or computer searching expertise, and works reasonably well if you are interested in finding studies on a single topic, but manual searching has serious limitations and is time-consuming. Foremost of the limitations are that (a) you must search year-by-year (you cannot search across multiple years), (b) there is no option of combining topics; and (c) there is no ability to screen out irrelevant sources by age group, focus of the article, or type of article. You must go through each citation under the topic and try to determine by the title and any information provided whether the study addresses your clinical questions.

If manual searching is all that is available to you, you should combine it with careful gleaning of the reference lists of the studies you have been able to obtain for other relevant studies. If you start with an index search of recent years and find one or two relevant studies, they will often point you to prior studies.

Appendix B. **Resources on the Internet**

CAVEAT

Resources and locations on the Internet change rapidly, so expect resources that are available today to have changed tomorrow, or perhaps not be available in the form in which you have formerly seen them. The information included in this appendix is based on what was available in late 1998.

LEARNING RESOURCES

For reading about accessing Internet resources, see:

Nicoll, L.H. (1998). *Nurses' Guide to the Internet,* 2nd ed. Philadelphia: Lippincott.

Sikorski, R., and Peters, R. (1997). Medical literature made easy: Querying databases on the Internet. *Journal of the American Medical Association, 277*:959–960.

Wayne-Doppke, J. (1997). *1997 Healthcare Guide to the Internet: An Annotated Listing of Internet Resources for the Healthcare Professional.* Santa Barbara, CA: COR Healthcare.

DATABASES

The Web site of the National Library of Medicine's main page provides links to several of the databases listed below. The site also provides links to many other potentially valuable sites for finding research studies on a particular topic.

Web site: http://www.nlm.nih.gov/

MEDLINE

Access: MEDLINE can be accessed on line without charge through PubMed or through Internet Grateful Med, both services of the National Library of Medicine. Abstracts (when available), related articles, links to full text versions at publishers' web sites (some free, some by subscription), and a system for ordering copies of documents are provided. Your hospital or university may have the MEDLINE database on an internal computer system, possibly with additional information such as local holding of journals.

Web site:http://www.ncbi.nlm.nih.gov/PubMed/

Web site for Internet Grateful Med: http://igm.nlm.nih.gov/

Producer: National Library of Medicine

CINAHL

Access: The CINAHL database can be accessed via CINAHL direct on the Internet or via Telnet options, both on a subscription basis. Technical support, search assistance, and document delivery are available. Your hospital library may have CINAHL available by CD ROM or by subscription without charge to you, so ask your librarian.

Web site: http://www.cinahl.com/

Producer: CINAHL Information Systems

HealthSTAR

Access: Available via "Grateful Med," an Internet site provided by the National Library of Medicine. Your hospital or university may have it available on an internal computer system.

Web site: http://igm.nlm.nih.gov/

Producer: National Library of Medicine

PsychINFO

Access: Available on the Internet through a commercial online vendor. May be available at your hospital or university library at no cost to you.

Web site: http://www.apa.org/psycinfo/

Producer: American Psychological Association

SciSearch and Social SciSearch

Access: May be available at your hospital or university library at no cost to you.

Web site: http://www.isinet.com/

Producer: Institute for Scientific Information

EMBASE

Access: May be available at your hospital or university library at no cost to you.

Web site: http://www.elsevier.com/

Producer: Elsevier Science

ERIC

Access: Available free on the Internet and in many public and academic libraries.

Web site: http://ericir.syr.edu/eric/

Producer: U.S. Department of Education

BIOETHICSLINE

Access: Available via "Grateful Med," an Internet site provided by the National Library of Medicine. Your hospital or university may have it available on an internal computer system.

Web site: http://www.nlm.nih.gov/

Producer: National Library of Medicine

CANCERLIT

Access: Available free on the Internet or through your library.
   Web site: http://cancernet.nci.nih.gov/
   Producer: National Cancer Institute

AIDSLINE

Access: Available on the Internet free through Internet Grateful Med or through your library.
   Web site: http:// igm.nlm.nih.gov/
   Producer: National Library of Medicine

LIBRARY CATALOGS

Directory of Library Catalogs (to obtain TELNET addresses of libraries around the world)
   Web site: http://library.usask.ca/hytelnet/sites1.html
National Library of Medicine (books, journals available at the NLM)
   Web site: http://www.nlm.nih.gov/
Virginia Henderson International Nursing Library (subscription services to: *Registry of Nursing Research* and *Online Journal of Nursing Synthesis for Nursing*)
   Web site: http://www.stti.iupui.edu/library

OTHER RESOURCES

Emory University List of Electronic Publications
   Web   site: http://www.gen.emory.edu/MEDWEB/keyword/electronic_ publications.html
HealthWeb: Collaborative effort of University of Michigan and Health Web Consortium
   Web site: http://www.healthweb.org/
U. S. Government documents
   Web site: http://www.access.gpo.gov/
UMI Document Delivery Services (Dissertations and other documents)
   Web site: http://www.umi.com/

INTERNET RESOURCES FOR EVIDENCE-BASED HEALTH CARE

Agency for Health Care Policy and Research
   Key guidelines, heavily evidence-based. Produced by U.S. Government.
   http://www.chcpr.gov/clinic/
American College of Physicians
   Information about ACP Journal Club, EBM Journal, and clinical guidelines.
   http://www.acponline.org

Bandolier
Full test reviews in easy-to-use subject format.
http://www.jr2.ox.ac.uk/bandolier/
Best Practice Network
Shares evaluated contributed practices, offers discussion groups, fosters innovative problem solving, and provides resource lists. A collaborative effort of professional health related organizations.
http://www.best4health.org
The Cochrane Collaboration
"Preparing, maintaining and promoting the accessibility of systematic reviews of the effects of healthcare interventions."
http://linux.chpt.es/cochrane/default.html
Database of Abstracts of Reviews of Effectiveness (DARE)
Full text abstracts in searchable format.
http://nhscrd.york.ac.uk/
Evidence-Based Care Home Page
Evidence-Based Informatics Project at McMaster University, Ontario, Canada.
http://hiru.hirunet.mcmaster.ca/ebm/
Netting the Evidence: A ScHARR Introduction to Evidence-Based Practice on the Internet
Provides a list of evidence-based medicine resources available on the Internet. Produced by University of Sheffield (UK), School of Health & Related Research (ScHARR).
http://www.med.unr.edu/medlib/netting.html
POEMS (Patient Oriented Evidence that Matters)
Reviews updated monthly, associated with Journal of Family Practice.
http://jfp.msu.edu/

SELECTED JOURNAL RESOURCES ON EVIDENCE-BASED HEALTH CARE

ACP Journal Club
Bimonthly, published by the American College of Physicians–American Society of Internal Medicine.
http://www.acponline.org/
Evidence-Based Health Policy & Management
Quarterly, published by Churchill Livingstone. Focused on policy rather than patient level.
orders@edinburgh.rsh.pearson-pro.com
Evidence-Based Medicine
Bimonthly, co-publication of the BMJ Publishing Group and the American College of Physicians–American Society of Internal Medicine
http://www.bmjpg.com/

Evidence-Based Mental Health
Quarterly, co-publication of the BMJ Publishing Group and the Royal College of Psychiatrists (UK).
http://www.bmjpg.com/
Evidence-Based Nursing
Quarterly, co-publication of the BMJ Publishing Group and the RCN Publishing Company, with support from the support of the Health Information Research Unit, McMaster University.
http://www.bmjpg.com/
User Guides to the Medicine Literature
A collection of articles published in the Journal of the American Medical Association on applying evidence-based medicine.
http://www.shef.ac.uk/~scharr/ir/userg.html

HEALTH CARE-ORIENTED INTERNET DIRECTORIES

MedWeb
http://www.emory.edu/whscl/medweb.html
Medical Matrix: Guide to Internet Clinical Medicine Resources
http://www.medmatrix.org/index.asp
HealthWeb
http:www.healthweb.org/
Yahoo—Health
http://www.yahoo.com/health

SEARCH ENGINES

AltaVista
http://www.altavista.com
Excite
http://www.excite.com/
Infoseek
http://www.infoseek.com/

Appendix C. **Example: Measures of Clinical Significance**

Data

In an experimental rehabilitation group, 64.2 percent of the patients returned to work within six months. In another group receiving standard care, only 48.4 percent of the patients did.

Calculations (working with positive outcome)

ARI (absolute rate of improvement)
    = rate of experimental group minus rate of control group
    = 64.2% − 48.4% = 15.8%
NNT (number needed to treat)
    = the inverse of ARI or 1/ARI
    = 1/.158 = 6.3 (round off to 6)
RB (relative benefit is the positive form of relative risk)
    = ratio of experimental group rate to control group rate
        (1 being equal risk for both groups)
    = 64.2/48.4 = 1.33.
RIR (relative improvement rate is the positive form of relative risk rate)
    = ratio of absolute improvement to the rate of return to
        work of the control group
    = [64.2 − 48.4]/48.4 = .33 = 33%

Interpretations

ARI: the difference in return to work rates between the experimental treatment and the standard care group was 15.8 percent.

NNT: the number of persons who would need to be treated with the experimental rehabilitation approach in order to achieve one additional case of return to work over what would be realized using standard treatment is 6.

RB: the relative benefit of the experimental treatment of 1.33 means that the experimental group return to work rate was 33 percent better than the rate of the control group (1 = equal benefit; >1 = greater benefit; and <1 = less benefit).

RIR: the relative rate of improvement of 0.33 or 33 percent means that the increased benefit achieved by the experimental group was a 33 percent improvement in relation to the rate experienced by the control group.

COMPARISON OF THE MEASURES OF CLINICAL SIGNIFICANCE

There are advantages and disadvantages to the portrayal of clinical significance by each of the measures. The disadvantage of RR and RRR is that they do not reflect the magnitude of the absolute treatment benefit, but

Table C–1. **Examples of Large and Small Treatment Effects**

Absolute Risk Improvement (ARI)	Numbers Needed to Treat (NNT)	Relative Benefit (RB)
Large effect (per example)		
$64.2\% - 48.4\% = 15.8\%$	$1/15.8\% = 1/0.158 = 6.3$	$64.2\%/48.4\% = 1.33$
Small effect		
$6.42\% - 4.84\% = 1.58\%$	$1/1.58\% = 1/0.0158 = 63.3$	$6.42\%/4.84\% = 1.33$

rather portray it relative to the control group result, which may hide the magnitude of the treatment effect (Sackett et al., 1997). Table C–1 displays the calculation of three measures of treatment effect using the rehabilitation example results, but also gives an example with a small treatment effect (one-tenth of the original example) to show how the magnitude of the treatment effect is reflected in the ARI and NNT but is masked in the RB (and it follows in the RIR).

The practitioner relying on the relative benefit measure of clinical significance would have a sense of the relative rate of improved return to work but would have no sense of how much the actual difference between the two approaches was. Although each of these measures provides a slightly different clinical portrayal of the benefits of the experimental rehabilitation approach, most sources recommend using the absolute risk reduction and the numbers needed to treat, as they incorporate both baseline risk and the magnitude of risk reduction (Laupacis, Sackett, and Roberts, 1988; Sackett, Richardson, Rosenberg, and Haynes, 1997).

References

Laupacis, A., Sackett, D.L., and Roberts, R.S. (1988). An assessment of clinically useful measures of the consequences of treatment. *The New England Journal of Medicine, 318,* 1728–1733.

Sackett, D.L., Richardson, W.S., Rosenberg, W., and Haynes, R.B. (1997). *Evidence-based Medicine: How to practice & teach EBM.* New York: Churchill Livingstone.

Appendix D. **Confidence Intervals Around the Difference Between Two Group Means**

CALCULATION

1. Calculate the standard error (SE) of the difference of the means SE (diff):

$$SE\ (diff) = \sqrt{\frac{(n_1 - 1)\ s^2_1 + (n_2 - 1)s^2_2}{n_1 + n_2 - 2} \times \left(\frac{1}{n_1} + \frac{1}{n_2}\right)}$$

s = standard deviation for that group

2. Calculate the 95% confidence interval (CI):*

95% CI = mean difference ± (2 × SE(diff))

WARMING EXAMPLE

This warming example is taken from Chapter 7 (Guiffre et al., 1991). Point estimates reported: mean minutes to 36°C (standard deviation)
blankets   153.1″ (77.8″)
warm air   112.2″ (52.3″)
difference   40.9″

1. Calculation of SE (diff)

$$SE\ (diff) = \sqrt{\frac{(29 - 1)\ (52.3)^2 + (31 - 1)\ (77.8)^2}{31 + 29 - 2} \times \left(\frac{1}{29} + \frac{1}{31}\right)}$$

= 17.23

2. Calculation of 95%CI

CI = 40.9″ ± (2 × 17.23″)
CI = 6.44″ to 75.36″

N.B. When a mean followed by a plus and minus sign (e.g., $x = 99 \pm 8.83$) is provided in a report, the numerical value after the sign is most often a standard deviation, which is not the same as a standard error of the

---

*Assumes: independent samples, approximately normal distribution, similar standard deviations in both groups, and degrees of freedom greater than 40. The confidence coefficient, which in this example is 2, will vary with the sample size; it is derived from the t-distribution for $N_1 + N_2 - 2$ degrees of freedom.

difference in the means. The standard deviations of each group are used to calculate the standard error of the difference in the means, and then the standard error of the difference in means is used in the calculation of the 95% confidence interval.

Appendix E. **Example: Appraisal of a Single Study**

APPRAISAL QUESTIONS FOR A SINGLE STUDY USING A DESCRIPTIVE DESIGN

Study Citation

Ooi, W. L., Barrett, S., Hossain, M., Kelley-Gagnon, M., and Lipsitz, L. A. (1997). Patterns of orthostatic blood pressure change and their clinical correlates in a frail, elderly population. *Journal of American Medical Association*, 277:299–304.

Synopsis

What was the problem or issue being studied?

Patterns of orthostatic blood pressure change and their correlates in the frail elderly.

Was there one main variable of interest or several? If one, list the features of that variable. If there were several variables of interest, list them.

Patterns of orthostatic blood pressure was the main variable. Aspects that were described included: supine systolic blood pressure (sbp) before breakfast, standing sbp at 1 min and 3 min before and after breakfast and lunch. Correlates examined included: patient profile information, co-morbidity, and medication taken.

Was there a clearly defined group of participants? Were subgroups of the sample compared?
What two or more distinct populations were compared?

Participants were persons > 60 yrs who were able to stand for a least 1 min and who were not expected to die or be discharged within 3 months.

Sample was subsequently divided into four groups: no orthostatic hypotension (oh), isolated oh, variable oh, persistent oh; the four groups were then compared in terms of profile, supine sbp before breakfast, co-morbidity, and medications.

Was the sample followed over time or was a cross-sectional design used?

Not applicable

If the study used the survey method, how was the sample of contacts selected?
What percentage of the contacts responded or participated?
How were the data collected?

Training and monitoring of nurses taking bp readings were done, procedures specifically spelled out, other information obtained from patients directly, from patients' charts, and from the Minimum Data Set of the nursing facility. BP taken supine before breakfast, standing before and after breakfast and lunch with readings taken at 1" and 3" after standing.

How were the data analyzed?

Descriptive statistics were compiled, but a prediction model was also generated. Predictive model was generated after controlling for CVD and non-CVD morbidity. Comparative data on four groups were very complete.

What were the important findings?

- 52% had oh at least once

- 14% had persistent oh (at all 4 times)

- persistent oh more prevalent in those >80 yrs

- oh most prevalent before breakfast (27%)

- bp reduction greater at 1" than at 3"

- Elevated supine sbp before breakfast, lightheadedness, anti-parkinson's disease medications, male gender, low body mass index, independence in activities are associated with oh.

Credibility Profile

Were all the important features of the main variable examined?

Two concerns: (1) They didn't control for timing of hypotensive medication administration; (2) they didn't extend standing bp readings into evening hours.

If there were several variables, was their selection well justified?

Not justified but are the ones commonly considered. Rationale for inclusion of body mass index, and medication categories not provided.

Were the variables of interest well defined? Is it clear how they were measured?

Yes, the measurements of the main ones were specifically described; some patient characteristic variables not defined, e.g., dementia, mood distress, depression (not a big issue).

Are the participants (or respondents) representative of the target population? (Random sampling from the population and a high participation/response rate are the best assurances of representativeness.)

Not clear how many failed to meet ability to stand for 1" criteria or how many persons refused to participate. As a result it is not completely clear to whom the results can be generalized.

If a survey, was any attempt made to consider the issue of the extent to which the respondents resemble the target population?

If a survey, was the interview schedule or questionnaire thoughtfully constructed, pilot tested and revised?

Was the data thoroughly analyzed?

Yes. Study title sounded like it would be a correlational study, but most findings were descriptive in nature. Would have liked some clinical significance measures provided.

How do these findings compare to other findings in the field?

Findings are consistent with other findings I have seen except for the issue of finding a lower incidence of drop in sbp after lunch. Could be related to different population (i.e., able to stand) and sbp not taken as often after meal completed as in the other studies.

OVERALL, ARE THE FINDINGS CREDIBLE? Yes _____ No _____

Clinical Significance Profile

Do I think the incidence, prevalence, distribution, patterns, trends, and interrelations of variables are clinically meaningful in size and importance?

- Number of persons with dizziness/lightheadedness on standing was remarkably different in the no oh and the persistent oh groups (17% for no oh group versus 37% for persistent oh group).

- Of person with supine sbp ≥ 160 after breakfast, 32% experienced dizziness/lightheadedness, whereas of those with supine sbp < 140, only 18% experienced these symptoms.

Relative risk of symptoms based on this data: RR = 0.18/0.32 = 0.56. Therefore, persons with BP < 140 are 56% as likely to experience dizziness/lightheadedness as those with sbp ≥ 160.

Conclusion: low supine sbp decreases likelihood of these experiences.

- Incidence of oh on standing before breakfast = 27%; after breakfast = 23% (ARR = 4.2%, RR = .85); after lunch = 21% (RR = .77).

Conclusion: postprandial risk less than before breakfast risk.

- Number of persons on antipsychotic medications (8% for no oh group, 15% for persistent oh group) and on anti-Parkinson's disease medications (5% for oh group, 13% for persistent oh group).

- Multiple co-morbidity also was different across groups (38% in no oh group, 49% in persistent oh group).

Are the differences between subgroups or between populations large enough to make a clinical difference?

The incidence and predictive value of the supine, before breakfast sbp are striking and may be very important, but the fact is we don't have supine, before breakfst sbp readings on many people. For office patients, would need to know what the correlation is between supine, before breakfast readings and office readings to use as a predictor. The RR for dizziness/ lightheadedness with supine sbp < 140 is impressive.

Are the important results present in a large proportion of the participants/respondents?

Yes, an overall prevalence rate of 52% for oh is sizable. Also 21% had supine sbp ≥ 160, 32% of which had oh symptoms.

ARE THE FINDINGS CLINICALLY MEANINGFUL? Yes __X__ No _____

Applicability Profile

Deferred as appraising collective findings on three studies.

To what groups of patients or situations can I extend these findings with confidence?

How effective is my current practice? On what rationale is my current practice based?

How *could* I change my practice based on these findings? Would this be a substantial, incremental, or soft change?

If I changed my practice in this way, could patients be subjected to potential harm, risk, or unreasonable effort?

Are there any organization, logistical, cost, or time barriers to changing my practice? Could they be overcome?

SHOULD I CHANGE MY PRACTICE BASED ON THESE FINDINGS? Yes _____ No _____

How should I go about making the change?

Once I change my practice, how will I know if patients have benefited?

Appendix F. **Example: Collective Findings Table**

Collective Findings Table Topic: postprandial orthostatic hypotension

Author(s) and Date	Question and/or Variables	Study Design/Sample Size and Profile	Findings (Indicate if Clinically Significant)
Ooi et al., 1997 sbp = systolic blood pressure oh = orthostatic hypotension = reduction of >20 mm Hg in all three studies	What is the pattern of orthostatic bp changes and their clinical determinants? Variables: frequency of oh, time of day, systolic bp before breakfast, lightheadedness on standing, gender, medication bp taken 4 times/day at 1" and 3" after standing	Frail elderly in 45 nursing homes n = 911 Aged 60 or older able to stand for 1"	50% had oh at least once 14% had persistent oh persistent oh more prevalent in those >80 years oh most prevalent before breakfast (27%) than after meals bp decline greater at 1" than at 3" elevated supine sbp before breakfast, lightheadedness, anti-Parkinson medications, male gender, low body mass index and independence in activities are associated with oh
Aronow & Ahn, 1994 pp = postprandial	Obtain baseline data regarding pp decreases in sbp	Elderly in long-term care facility n = 499	

	Does a marked decrease in sbp correlate with higher incidence of falls and syncope? Variables: timing of maximal decrease, syncope, falls, medications bp taken sitting at 15" intervals × 5 and at 120" after lunch	mean age = 80 years, 71% female, 66% white, 27% black, 68% ambulatory, 32% wheelchair bound	24% had pp sbp decrease >22 mm Hg 56% had max decrease at 45"–60" after lunch, greater reductions in persons with: hx of syncope, hx of falls, persons on certain meds (SCE inhibitors, calcium channel blockers, nitrates, and others)
Vaitkevicius, et al., 1991	What is frequency and importance of pp reductions in sbp? bp taken sitting or in bed if bed-bound at 15" intervals × 5 after lunch	Debilitated, elderly in nursing home n = 113 volunteers mean age = 78, 14% ambulatory, 73% female, 71% had cv diagnosis, 50% had neuro dx, 54% on drugs that act on cns	36% had pp sbp reductions of >20 mm Hg Max decrease at 45"–60" after meal greater reductions in persons with hx of syncope, on vasodilating drugs, with higher premeal sbp, and with dependent leg position

References for Collective Findings Table

Aronow, W. S., and Ahn, C. (1994). Postprandial hypotension in 499 elderly persons in a long-term health care facility. *Journal of the American Geriatrics Society, 42:*930–932.

Ooi, W. L., Barrett, S., Hossain, M., Kelley-Gagnon, M., and Lipsitz, L. A. (1997). Patterns of orthostatic blood pressure change and their clinical correlates in a frail, elderly population. *Journal of American Medical Association, 277:*1299–1304.

Vaitkevicius, P. V., Esserwein, D. M., Maynard, A. K., O'Connor, F. C., and Fleg, J. L. (1991). Frequency and importance of postprandial blood pressure reduction in elderly nursing-home patients. *Annals of Internal Medicine, 115:*865–870.

Appendix G. **Example: Appraisal of Collective Evidence**

> ### Appraisal Questions for Collective Evidence Regarding Health or Illness Factors

Question:

Do the elderly experience orthostatic blood pressure drops after meals that might precipitate syncope or falls? [Note: based on three (3) studies only, not on all findings relevant to the question. (Ooi et al., 1997; Aronow & Ahn, 1994; Vaitkevicius et al., 1991)]

Across-Studies Synthesis

What individual factors are supported as important by more than one study?

• Incidence of orthostatic hypotension (defined in all studies as reduction in sbp >20 mmHg) is between 24% and 50%; incidence highest in sample of patients who could stand.

• Three studies established reduction in sbp does occur after lunch.

• Two studies found most persons experienced maximum reduction in sbp 45"–60" after completing lunch.

What relationships between factors are supported by more than one study?

• Three studies established that oh is associated with history of syncope or falls or lightheadedness on standing.

• All three studies established association with medications but with different categories.

Of the individual factor findings and relationship findings that were supported by more than one study, which ones did I consider clinically significant?

The association of oh with hx of syncope or falls or experience of lightheadedness or dizziness.

Is there a compelling finding from just one study for a factor, or association? Why do I consider it compelling?

• Ooi found: incidence of oh associated with high supine sbp before breakfast,

persistent oh associated with age > 80 yrs,

found greatest oh reduction before breakfast.

• Ooi's findings are compelling because he looked at sbp across the day and obtained supine, before breakfast, baseline readings.

What findings are inconsistent across studies?

The findings regarding after lunch oh are inconsistent with two studies finding 24% and 36%, but Ooi finding 21%; difference could be due to the number of times the orthostatic sbp reading was taken after the meal. The findings regarding medications are not consistent, as each study examined different categories.

What findings are contradictory across studies?

The findings regarding ACE inhibitors are contradictory (Ooi versus A & A).

Is there a theory that explains how the factors work together to contribute to the behavior, situation, or process of interest? Do the findings support a particular theory that explains the experience, process, behavior, or situation? Does my conceptual map help make sense of the dynamics that bring about the behavior or situation or cause the process to play out in a certain way?

This work is largely empirical, but there are studies examining physiological mechanisms associated with oh.

Were any of the studies conducted on a sample with characteristics similar to the patient I have in mind or the patients I see?

These patients were all in extended care situations, but Ooi had people who could stand and Aronow & Ahn had 68% ambulatory persons; ages similar to patients J see. Data is on patients who are probably more debilitated and less active than patients J see in primary care, but similar to my nursing home patients.

WHAT FINDINGS ABOUT THIS SITUATION, BEHAVIOR, OR PROCESS EARN MY CONFIDENCE BECAUSE THEY ARE WELL SUPPORTED BY THE RESEARCH EVIDENCE?

Between 24% and 50% of elderly in long-term care facilities experience at least one episode of oh during the day. All three studies indicate there is a postprandial sbp drop after lunch in many elderly, but it may not be as severe or as prevalent as a before breakfast drop (O). Oh is more likely in those with high sbp (O and V), and those on cardiovascular medications (A & A and V) and possibly anti-Parkinson's disease and antipsychotic medications (O); it is also more prevalent in those age 80 and older and possibly in those who are ambulatory (O and V). Findings from all three studies associate these symptoms with oh: dizziness/lightheadedness (O); hx of syncope (V and A & A); and hx of falls (A & A).

Change in Practice?

On what theory or view of the experience, behavior, situation, or process is my current practice based? How does that basis compare to the theory or view the research evidence provides/supports?

I wasn't sure if there really was a high association between oh and symptoms, although I suspected it was likely due to impaired baroreflex performance with aging. I didn't know if there were certain times when oh was more likely to occur although I had heard the theory of after meals. The relationship of oh to CV medications is not surprising to me.

If I were to use the findings in which I have confidence, specifically how would my practice be changed?

• I would think more in terms of the profile of persons whom I should advise about the possibility of oh and associated symptoms, and pay most attention to those over age 80 with sbp >160, and on CV drugs, anti-Parkinson's drugs, or antipsychotic drugs. Treat hypertension in all elderly persons with oh symptoms and sbp >160.

• For nursing home patients: I would ask for supine and standing (after 1") bp readings once weekly before breakfast and 45" after lunch on patients at greatest risk. (Remember to discontinue after one month or stability and then just request periodically.)

Would making this change involve a substantial, incremental, or soft change?

Incremental change to more consistent treating of persons with sbp >160 and oh symptoms. I now request orthostatic signs on some patients at nursing home, but these findings would help me target those requests better.

Would inclusion of the finding(s) into practice impose any burden or risk on the patient, on me, or on the agency?

Might scare some patients but nothing beyond that. Modest increased work for nursing home staff.

SHOULD I CHANGE MY PRACTICE BASED ON THIS EVIDENCE? Yes _____ No _____

How should I go about making the change?

Introduce the issue into conversations with patients. Explain rationale for oh signs to nursing home staff, leave copy of Ooi et al. study for them to read.

Once I change my practice, how will I know if patients have benefited?

I'll keep an office log of those > age 80 with office sbp above 160 whose hpertension I treat. Record: office lying SBP, office standing-after-lying sbp, oh symptoms at home. Analyze after 25 patients to determine incidence of symptoms and office oh (should be less than 25%).

Appendix H. **Example: Appraisal of an Integrative Research Review**

Appraisal Questions for an Integrative Research Review

Citation:

Eichorst, A.M., Janken, J.K., and Mullen, T.M. (1997). The therapeutic value of cranberries in treating and preventing urinary tract infections. The Online Journal of Knowledge Synthesis for Nursing, 4, document 2, April 29, 1997.

Synopsis

What topic or question did the integrative review address?

The therapeutic value of cranberry juice (cj) in treating urinary tract infections (UTJs).

Examined: acidification of urine, inhibiting of adherence of bacteria to bladder cells, effectiveness in preventing and treating UTJs, and enhancement of antibiotic effectiveness.

How were potential, relevant research reports identified?

Authors state they used MEDLJNE EXPRESS 1966–1995, English language journals with search terms: cranberry juice, cranberries, bacteriuria, urine acidity, and urinary tract infection. Seem to have identified eight studies via this search; must have also used reference searches to obtain other study reports.

What determined if a research report was included in the analysis or not?

Can't tell; generally method by which these studies came to be included in the analysis is not described.

How many studies were included in the analysis?

16 (oldest 1914, most recent 1994)

What research methods were used in the studies included in the analysis?

A wide variety: animal studies, in vitro studies, case studies, descriptive, quasi-experimental, and one randomized experimental study.

What were the important and consistent findings?

• Two studies support the theory that ingestion of a cranberry product results in acidic urine, the other eight do not.

• In vitro, in mice, and in vivo studies provide consistent support for the theory that cranberry juice inhibits the adherence of bacteria to bladder cells.

• The only randomized, controlled, longitudinal study of cranberry juice effectiveness found that bacteriuria and pyuria were significantly less in the cranberry beverage group (15%) than in the placebo group (28%) beginning after one month and continuing for the four months of the study.

• In vivo and clinical study evidence to support hypothesis that certain antibiotics are more effective in an acidic environment, but no evidence to suggest that cranberry juice can produce the necessary acidification.

What were the analyst's conclusions?

One clinical trial and several descriptive reports suggest that drinking cranberry juice is an effective deterrent to UTIs. Research evidence indicates that cranberries interfere with the ability of bacteria to adhere to bladder cells. No evidence to suggest that cranberry ingestion enhances antibiotic effectiveness.

Credibility Profile

Was the topic clearly defined and clinically meaningful?

Yes, questions were specific and targeted both the physiological mechanism and clinical effectiveness.

Was the search for potential reports broad and unbiased?

The report reads like the review was inclusive of all studies on the topic, but can't be sure of this because few details regarding the search were provided.

Were the characteristics of the studies displayed or discussed in sufficient detail?

Excellent display and thorough discussion of study specifics by clinical questions.

Is there truly an integration of findings or merely a reporting of separate findings?

The integration across studies addressed limits and strengths of the study designs as well as the amount and consistency of findings.

Do the overall findings accurately reflect the findings from the individual studies?

Yes, definitely congruent.

Which overall findings were consistently well supported and which were less well supported? What, if anything, could explain the differences in results from study to study?

There is limited support for all questions, but the question of acidification of urine is the least well supported. One randomized study does support effectiveness of cj in preventing UTJs after one month of ingesting 300 ml of cj per day with no evidence to the contrary.

ARE THE CONCLUSIONS OF THE INTEGRATION CREDIBLE? Yes __X__ No _____

Clinical Significance

Do the conclusions resonate with what I see in everyday practice?

J hear many anecdotal claims for the effectiveness of cj, but details vary widely and are mostly lacking.

What findings are sizable enough and consistent enough that the conclusions are likely to hold up in everyday practice?

• For the one randomized study: incidence of bacteriuria is 15% for cj group and 28% for placebo group.

• The measures of clinical significance on these findings are as follows:

Relative risk = 15/28 = 0.54. Therefore, persons taking cj as in this study would have 54% as much risk of acquiring bacteriuria as persons not taking it.

Numbers needed to treat to prevent one less case of bacteriuria = 1/13 = 7.7 cases.

• Conclusion: Jngesting cj has a high likelihood of producing a clinical benefit and does so without any known risk to the patient.

Applicability Profile

Are my patients similar to any of those studied? Are they similar to those in a particular study? Was there anything of note in the results for samples or subsamples that are most like my patient(s)?

The randomized study was conducted on 153 elderly women, which represents one of the groups which asked me about cj effectivenss. The other group is sexually active women with recurrent UTJs. J would be hesitant to extend these findings to the latter group. Jt's not clear from the review how many in sample had bacteriuria at the beginning of the study or how many had hx of UTJs. J need to obtain this study report!

Are the outcomes achieved of value to me or my patient(s)?

The linkage between cj and UTI symptoms is not established by this study, thus cj ingestion may or may not translate to improvement or no onset of symptoms.

What were the key features of the approach or intervention?

300 ml of cranberry juice sweetened with saccharin ingestion per day. (Is the saccharin a factor?)

Am I able to safely and effectively use the approach or intervention described?

Yes, easy to describe.

Are the findings and conclusions impressive enough to warrant trying them in your practice?

I think so, especially with elderly women, but not clear if it just prevents bacteriuria or also reduces frequency of UTIs in women with history of frequent UTIs.

Are there any organizational, logistical, cost, or time barriers to incorporating this approach into my practice? Could they be overcome?

No barriers really. 300 ml/day of cj is an inexpensive, easy-to-enact recommendation and carries no risk.

What changes, additions, training or purchases would be needed to start using this approach?

None.

SHOULD I CHANGE MY PRACTICE BASED ON THESE FINDINGS? Yes __X__ No _____

Once I change my practice, how will I know if the change has improved the care I give?

Identify five to ten elderly women with hx of UTIs who are not ingesting cj on a regular basis; then strongly recommend 300 ml cj/day to them; and at each visit, get urine culture and ask about adherence to recommendation and symptoms of UTI (document in record). After 1 year look at charts and compare frequency of before and after in those who were compliant.

Appendix I. **Appraisal Forms**

This appendix contains a full set of appraisal forms which may be enlarged and copied for reader use. They are listed here for easy reference.

Appraisal forms for the findings of single studies:
1. Non-experimental, qualitative methods
2. Non-experimental, descriptive, survey designs
3. Non-experimental, correlational designs
4. Experimental designs
5. Quasi-experimental designs

Collective findings table

Appraisal forms for collective evidence regarding:
1. Patient experiences
2. Health or illness factors
3. Therapies and interventions
4. Potential assessment tools

Appraisal forms for state-of-the-science summaries:
1. Meta-analysis
2. Integrative research review
3. Research-based practice guideline

Appraisal of the Findings of a Single, Original Study Using a Non-experimental, Qualitative Method

---

Study Citation

Synopsis

What experience, adaptive process, social process, or environment was studied?

What was the research question?

What kinds of people or situations were studied?

How was data collected?

What procedures were used to transform the data into more general categories or themes?

What are the findings? What form did the findings take (a description, a conceptual explanation, a theory, a model)?

Credibility Profile

Were participants allowed to describe their experiences and points of view in their own words? *AND/OR* were extensive and carefully documented observations conducted? *AND/OR* were patients' diaries, transcripts of dialogue, or historical records systematically analyzed?

Were participants' quotes and/or vivid descriptions provided in the report?

Were sufficient cases, situations, or narrative examined to convince me that a potentially generalizable pattern was identified?

Do the researcher's conclusions flow logically from the raw data?

Did the researcher confirm the interpretations/findings with any participants?

How does this finding compare to other findings in the field?

OVERALL, IS THE FINDING CREDIBLE? Yes _____ No _____

Clinical Significance Profile

Do the findings resonate with how I have experienced the reality they are portraying?

Do these findings suggest a way of viewing a patient's situation that is significantly more sensitive, more complete, or more adequate than how I have previously thought about the situation?

Was the result present in a majority of the cases and are impressive as capturing an important aspect of the experience, process, or situation?

IS THE FINDING CLINICALLY SIGNIFICANT? Yes _____ No _____

Applicability Profile

How effective is my current practice? On what rationale is my current practice based?

To what groups of patients or situations can I extend these findings with confidence?

How *could* I change my practice based on these findings? Would this be a substantial, incremental, or soft change?

If I changed my practice in this way could patients be subjected to potential harm or risk?

Are there any organizational, logistical, cost, or time barriers to changing my practice? Could they be overcome?

SHOULD I CHANGE MY PRACTICE BASED ON THIS FINDING? Yes _____ No _____

How should I go about making the change?

Once I change my practice, how will I know if patients have benefited?

Appraisal of the Findings of a Single, Original Study Using a Non-experimental Descriptive Design

---

Study Citation

Synopsis

What was the question or issue being studied?

Was there one main variable of interest or several? If one, list the features of that variable that were examined. If there were several variables of interest, list them.

Was there a clearly defined group of participants? Were subgroups of the sample compared?

OR what two or more distinct populations were compared?

Was the sample followed over time or was a cross-sectional design used?

If the study used survey methods, how was the sample of contacts selected?

What percentage of the contacts responded or participated?

How were the data collected?

How were the data analyzed?

What were the important findings?

Credibility Profile

Were all the important features of the main variable examined?

If there were several variables, was their selection well justified?

Were the variables of interest well defined? Is it clear how they were measured?

Are the participants (or respondents) representative of the target population? (Random sampling from the population and a high participation/ response rate are the best assurances of representativeness.)

If a survey, was any attempt made to consider the issue of the extent to which the respondents resemble the target population?

If a survey, was the interview schedule or questionnaire thoughtfully constructed, pilot tested, and revised?

Were the data thoroughly analyzed?

How does this finding compare to other findings in the field?

OVERALL, IS THE FINDING CREDIBLE? Yes _____ No _____

Clinical Significance Profile

Do I think the incidence, prevalence, distribution, patterns, trends, and interrelations of variables are clinically meaningful in size and importance?

Are the differences between subgroups or between populations large enough to make a clinical difference?

Are the important results present in a large proportion of the participants/respondents?

Is THE FINDING CLINICALLY MEANINGFUL? Yes _____ No _____

Applicability Profile

To what groups of patients or situations can I extend this finding with confidence?

How effective is my current practice? On what rationale is my current practice based?

How *could* I change my practice based on these findings? Would this be a substantial, incremental, or soft change?

If I changed my practice in this way, could patients be subjected to potential harm, risk, or unreasonable effort?

Are there any organizational, logistical, cost, or time barriers to changing my practice? Could they be overcome?

SHOULD I CHANGE MY PRACTICE BASED ON THIS FINDING? Yes _____ No _____

How should I go about making the change?

Once I change my practice, how will I know if patients have benefited?

Appraisal of the Findings of a Single, Original Study Using Non-experimental, Correlational Design

---

Study Citation

Synopsis

What was the general topic or question of interest?

What variables were studied?

Was the strength of relationship between variables examined or were some used to predict others? Was a model composed of many variables tested?

What population does the sample represent?

How large was the sample?

What correlations/associations between variables were statistically significant?

Credibility Profile

Are the reasons for studying the variables plausible and/or connected to previous theoretical and/or empirical work in the field?

Were the research variables translated into measurements in logically sound ways?

Do the measuring instruments used have established reliability and validity?

Was the sample selected in a way that convinces me that it is representative of the target population?

Is the sample size large enough to detect associations (i.e., sufficient statistical power)?

If many correlations, or associations, were calculated, was there an adjustment to avoid chance results of significant correlations (Type I error)?

Were the sample's scores distributed across a wide range of possible scores on the measuring instrument?

Did the researcher indicate if there was a search for outliers and if they were removed prior to computing the correlation coefficient?

How does this finding compare to other findings in the field?

OVERALL, ARE THE FINDINGS CREDIBLE? Yes _____ No _____

Clinical Significance Profile

In descriptive correlational studies, how strong is the association found between the variables? What is the amount of co-influence, i.e., what is the r^2 level? Does it indicate a strong or weak connection?

In predictive correlational studies, is the proportion of the outcome variable predicted by the independent variable(s) large enough to have practical meaning, i.e., what is the R^2 value? What variables have a large amount of influence on the outcome variable?

In model testing correlational studies, what proportion of the outcome variable is predicted by the other variables in the trimmed or revised model, i.e., what is its R^2 value? What pathways of influence are clinically important?

IS THE ASSOCIATION BETWEEN/AMONG VARIABLES CLINICALLY MEANINGFUL IN SIZE AND IMPORTANCE? Yes _____ No _____

Applicability Profile

To what groups of patients or situations can I extend this finding with confidence?

How *could* I change my practice based on this finding? Would this be a substantial, incremental, or soft change?

If I changed my practice in this way, could patients be subjected to potential harm or risk?

How effective is my current practice? On what rationale is my current practice based?

Are there any organizational, logistical, cost, or time barriers to changing my practice? How could they be overcome?

SHOULD I CHANGE MY PRACTICE BASED ON THESE FINDINGS? Yes _____ No _____

How should I go about making the change?

Once I change my practice, how will I know if patients have benefited?

Appraisal Questions for a Single, Original Study Using an
Experimental Design

Study Citation

Synopsis

What interventions, treatments, preventive services, or therapies were compared?

What outcomes were evaluated?

What populations were targeted?

How was the sample of participants acquired?

Were the participants truly randomly assigned to treatment groups?

What intervention delivery and data collection procedures were followed?

What measuring instruments were used? Do they have established validity and reliability?

What were the important findings?

Credibility Profile

Were providers, patients, and raters blind to the treatment each participant received?

If the treatment was administered over a lengthy period, were there checks to assure that it was consistently being administered in accordance with original specifications?

Were all participants who were originally randomized to a treatment group included in the data analysis? Were drop-out rates and failure to follow protocol rates reported and considered?

If differences were found

Could something other than the treatment variable have resulted in the groups having different outcomes?

Was there a check to determine if random assignment actually did evenly distribute confounding demographic and personal variables?

Other than the different treatments, were the groups treated equally?

If differences were found between subgroups, was the number of comparison tests done small in number or were the results adjusted for multiple tests?

If no differences were found

Could something in the way the study was done have resulted in the two groups having similar outcomes?

Was the sample large enough to detect a difference among the groups if one truly occurred? Was a power analysis done to determine sample size?

Were the treatments themselves different enough to create a real difference in outcomes?

Is the association between the treatment and the outcome(s) plausible based on other available knowledge and information?

How does this finding compare to other work in the field?

OVERALL, ARE THE FINDINGS CREDIBLE? Yes _____ No _____

Clinical Significance Profile

Note or calculate a measure of clinical significance for each result and deliberate on its clinical meaning.

IS THE RESULT CLINICALLY SIGNIFICANT? Yes _____ No _____

Applicability Profile

To what groups of patients or situations can I extend these findings with confidence?

Were there serious or annoying side effects?

Does the intervention subject the patient to any risks?

Was there inordinate effort required of the patients to use the experimental treatment?

How *could* I change my practice based on these findings? Would this be a substantial, incremental, or soft change?

If I changed my practice in this way, could patients be subjected to potential harm or risk?

How effective is my current practice? On what rationale is my current practice based?

Are there any organizational, logistical, cost, or time barriers to changing my practice? How could they be overcome?

SHOULD I CHANGE MY PRACTICE BASED ON THESE FINDINGS? Yes _____ No _____

How should I go about making the change?

Once I change my practice, how will I know if patients have benefited?

> ## Appraisal of the Findings of a Single, Original Study Using a Quasi-Experimental Design

Study Citation

Synopsis

What interventions, treatments, preventive services, or therapies were compared?

Was the intervention directly manipulated by the research team?

What form of intervention did the comparison group or control group receive?

What outcomes were evaluated?

What populations were targeted?

How were the participants assigned to treatment groups?

How long were the comparison groups followed?

What cause and effect relationships were hypothesized?

What are the findings?

Credibility Profile

Were providers, patients, and raters blind to the treatment each participant received?

If the treatment was administered over a lengthy period, were there checks to assure that it was consistently being administered in accordance with original specifications?

Were all participants who were originally randomized to a treatment group included in the data analysis? Were drop-out rates and failure to follow protocol rates reported and considered?

If differences were found

Could something other than the treatment variable have resulted in the two groups having different outcomes?

Was there a check to determine if random assignment actually did evenly distribute confounding demographic and personal variables?

Other than the different treatments, were the groups treated equally?

If differences were found between subgroups, was the number of comparison tests done small in number or were the results adjusted for multiple tests?

If no differences were found

Could something in the way the study was done have resulted in the two groups having similar outcomes?

Was the sample large enough to detect a difference among the groups if one truly occurred? Was a power analysis done to determine sample size?

Were the treatments themselves different enough to create a real difference in outcomes?

Is the association between the treatment and the outcome(s) plausible based on other available knowledge and information?

How does this finding compare to other findings in the field?

OVERALL, IS THIS FINDING CREDIBLE? Yes _____ No _____

Clinical Significance Profile

Note or calculate a measure of clinical significance for each result and deliberate on its clinical meaning.

IS THE RESULT CLINICALLY SIGNIFICANT? Yes _____ No _____

Applicability Profile

To what groups of patients or situations can I extend this finding with confidence?

Were there serious or annoying side effects? Was there inordinate effort required of the patients to use the experimental treatment?

How *could* I change my practice based on these findings? Would this be a substantial, incremental, or soft change?

If I changed my practice in this way, could patients be subjected to potential harm or risk?

How effective is my current practice? On what rationale is my current practice based?

Are there any organizational, logistical, cost, or time barriers to changing my practice? How could they be overcome?

SHOULD I CHANGE MY PRACTICE BASED ON THESE FINDINGS? Yes _____ No _____

How should I go about making the change?

Once I change my practice, how will I know if patients have benefited?

Collective Findings Table

Topic: _____

Author(s) & Date	Question and/or Variables	Study Design/Sample Size & Profile	Findings (indicate if Clinically Significant)

Appraisal Questions for Collective Evidence Regarding Patient Experiences

---

Across-Studies Syntheses

Note which findings describe the experience at a point in time and those which describe it over time.

Note which findings address the fine points or subtleties of an experience, and those that convey a better overall picture of the experience.

What findings are supported by more than one study?

Is there a compelling finding from just one study for an insight, factor, or association? Why do I consider it compelling?

What findings are outrightly contradictory from one study to another? Can these differences in findings be explained by differences in samples or research methods?

What findings resulted from studies using samples similar to the patient(s) with whom I will be using the findings?

Do any of the findings resonate with my experience more than others or provide a fresh view on the particular patient experience?

What findings related to this patient experience earn my confidence because they are well supported by the research evidence?

Change in Practice?

If I were to use the findings in which I have confidence, specifically what would I do differently?

Would making this change involve a substantial, incremental, or soft change?

Would inclusion of the finding(s) into practice impose any burden or risk on the patient, on me, or on the agency?

Would this inclusion be feasible practically and economically?

SHOULD I CHANGE MY PRACTICE BASED ON THIS EVIDENCE? Yes _____ No _____

How should I go about making the change?

Once I change my practice, how will I know if patients have benefited?

Appraisal Questions for Collective Evidence Regarding Health or Illness Factors

---

Across-Studies Syntheses

What individual factors are supported as important by more than one study?

What relationships between factors are supported by more than one study?

Of the individual factor findings and relationship findings that were supported by more than one study, which ones did I consider clinically significant?

Is there a compelling finding from just one study for a factor, or association? Why do I consider it compelling?

What findings are inconsistent from one study to another?

What findings are outrightly contradictory from one study to another? Can these differences in findings be explained by differences in samples or research methods?

Is there a theory that explains how the factors work together to contribute to the behavior, situation, or process of interest? *OR* Do the findings support a particular theory that explains the experience, process, behavior, or situation? *OR* Does my conceptual map help make sense of the dynamics that bring about the behavior or situation or cause the process to play out in a certain way?

Were any of the studies conducted on a sample with characteristics similar to the patient(s) I have in mind?

What findings about this situation, behavior, or process earn my confidence because they are well supported by the research evidence?

Change in Practice?

On what theory or view of the experience, behavior, situation, or process is my current practice based? How does that basis compare to the theory or view the research evidence provides/supports?

If I were to use the findings in which I have confidence, specifically how would my practice be changed?

Would making this change involve a substantial, incremental, or soft change?

Would inclusion of the finding(s) into practice impose any burden or risk on the patient, on me, or on the agency?

Would this inclusion be feasible practically and economically?

SHOULD I CHANGE MY PRACTICE BASED ON THIS EVIDENCE? Yes _____ No _____

How should I go about making the change?

Once I change my practice, how will I know if patients have benefited?

Appraisal Questions for Collective Evidence Regarding
Therapies and Interventions

Across-Studies Syntheses

How much variation was there in how the intervention was delivered across the studies?

How much variation was there in the outcomes studied across the studies?

What findings are supported by more than one study?

What findings are supported by just one study but are compelling. Why are they compelling?

What findings are inconsistent across studies?

What findings are outrightly contradictory across studies?

Note the levels of evidence from the various studies and the findings associated with them. Is a randomized clinical trial feasible? Are findings from one available?

Of the consistent findings, how many studies had a treatment effect that was clinically significant?

What outcome(s) is this intervention highly effective in bringing about?

What side effects, harm, or burden is associated with this intervention?

Is the evidence picture sufficiently complete (i.e., knowledge regarding: benefits, risks, burden, underlying mechanism, specifics of administration)?

COMBINING CONSISTENCY OF FINDINGS ACROSS STUDIES, LEVELS OF EVIDENCE AVAILABLE, CLINICAL SIGNIFICANCE OF THE FINDINGS, AND SIMILARITY AND DIFFERENCES IN SAMPLES, IN WHAT FINDINGS CAN I HAVE CONFIDENCE?

Change in Practice?

Is my patient similar to those in whom the intervention was studied? Is my patient similar to any of the subgroups of patients for whom the intervention was beneficial?

Does my patient value the outcomes this intervention is likely to produce?

Is the intervention, including the burdens it imposes and any risks accompanying it, acceptable to my patient and me?

Do my patient and I possess the knowledge and skills to safely and effectively use this intervention? What would be required to acquire them?

Is the intervention paid for by the reimbursement system with which the patient and I are associated?

Would using this intervention involve a substantial, incremental, or soft change?

SHOULD I CHANGE MY PRACTICE BASED ON THIS EVIDENCE? Yes _____ No _____

How should I go about making the change?

Once I change my practice, how will I know if patients have benefited?

Appraisal Questions for Collective Evidence Regarding a Potential Assessment Tool

---

Across-Studies Syntheses

Specifically, what was the instrument designed to measure?

How carefully was the instrument developed conceptually?

How many studies have evaluated the reliability, validity, sensitivity, and specificity of this instrument?

What do the authors of these studies have to say about these qualities of the instrument?

Has the instrument been found to be capable of detecting small but clinically significant differences in patient status?

How many of these studies were conducted on samples and applications similar to how we will be using the instrument?

What risks or harms may be associated with the use of this instrument?

COMBINING CONSISTENCY OF FINDINGS ACROSS STUDIES, LEVELS OF EVIDENCE AVAILABLE, CLINICAL SIGNIFICANCE OF THE FINDINGS, AND SIMILARITY AND DIFFERENCES IN SAMPLES, CAN WE HAVE CONFIDENCE THAT THIS INSTRUMENT PROVIDES QUALITY CLINICAL INFORMATION? Yes _____ No _____

Change in Practice?

How do we currently assess, evaluate, or measure the attribute this instrument measures?

In what ways are we dissatisfied with our current assessment tool/instrument?

How would adoption of the use of this instrument be an improvement over current practice?

In reading about how this instrument is used, can we see any reason why it might be unreliable, cumbersome, or difficult to use in our clinical setting (think of both patients and staff)?

Would adopting the instrument involve a substantial or incremental change?

Does our agency or practice have the resources to reliably use this instrument on an ongoing basis (i.e., equipment purchase and maintenance, personnel training, interpretation expertise)?

SHOULD WE CHANGE OUR PRACTICE BASED ON THIS EVIDENCE? Yes _____ No _____

Once we make the change in practice, how will we know if patients have benefited?

Appraisal of the Evidence From a Meta-Analysis

Citation

Synopsis

What was the question the meta-analysis set out to answer? What types or classes of interventions were compared? What outcomes were studied? What associations between variables were of interest?

How were potential, relevant research reports identified?

What determined if a research report was included in the analysis or not?

How many studies were included in each part of the analysis?

What mix of design types was used in the individual studies?

What measure of effect size was used, e.g., effect size statistic, treatment response rate, relative risk, numbers needed to treat?

What were the important findings?

What were the analysts' conclusions?

Credibility Profile

Was the research question clear and clinically meaningful?

Were the methods of the analysis reported in sufficient detail to enable a replication of the analysis?

Was the search for potential reports broad and unbiased?

Were inclusion or exclusion criteria explicitly set forth?

Was the credibility, i.e., scientific soundness, of the individual studies assessed? Was this decision made in a reliable and objective manner? Were seriously flawed studies eliminated from the analysis?

Was separate information provided for randomized and non-randomized studies?

ARE THE RESULTS CREDIBLE? Yes _____ No _____

Clinical Significance

How consistent were the results across studies, i.e., what percentage showed a treatment effect in the same direction? If quite variable, could the differences be explained by differences in populations, treatments, or outcomes?

Was there a clear, consistently found result regarding the efficacy of a particular treatment, either when compared to a placebo treatment or when compared to another treatment? Was a relationship between variables consistently found?

Was the overall effect size large, modest, or small? Was the effect size clinically meaningful?

Was the effect size for any subgroup of studies of interest to me large, modest, or small?

DO I THINK THE ASSOCIATION BETWEEN THE TREATMENT OR RISK FACTOR AND THE OUTCOME(S) IS LARGE ENOUGH TO MAKE A DIFFERENCE IN PATIENTS' WELL-BEING? Yes _____ No _____

Applicability Profile

Are the resulting benefits of the treatment/risk factor impressive vis-à-vis the risks and cost?

Are the outcomes achieved of value to my patient(s)?

Are the patients I treat, or the patient I am treating, similar to any of those included in the analysis?

Am I able to safely and effectively use this intervention?

Are there any organizational, logistical, financial, or time barriers to incorporating this intervention into my practice? How could they be overcome?

What changes, additions, training, or purchases would be needed to start using this intervention?

SHOULD I CHANGE MY PRACTICE BASED ON THESE FINDINGS? Yes _____ No _____

Once I change my practice, how will I know if the change has improved the care I give?

Appraisal of the Evidence From an Integrative Research Review

Citation

Synopsis

What topic or question did the integrative review address?

How were potential, relevant research reports identified?

What determined if a research report was included in the analysis or not?

How many studies were included in the analysis?

What research methods were used in the studies included in the analysis?

What were the important and consistent findings?

What were the analyst's conclusions?

Credibility Profile

Was the topic clearly defined and clinically meaningful?

Was the search for potential reports broad and unbiased?

Were the characteristics of the studies displayed or discussed in sufficient detail?

Is there truly an integration/synthesis of findings or merely a reporting of separate findings?

Do the overall findings accurately reflect the findings from all the individual studies?

What overall findings were consistently well supported and which were less well supported? What, if anything, could explain differences in results from study to study?

ARE THE CONCLUSIONS OF THE INTEGRATION CREDIBLE? Yes _____ No _____

Clinical Significance

Do the conclusions resonate with what I see in everyday practice?

Are the majority of the findings sizable enough, consistent enough, and well enough supported that the conclusions are likely to hold up in everyday practice?

Applicability Profile

Are my patients similar to any of those studied? Are they similar to those in a particular study? Was there anything of note in the results for samples or subsamples that are most like my patient(s)?

Are the outcomes achieved of value to me or my patient(s)?

What were the key features of the approach or intervention?

Am I able to safely and effectively use the approach or intervention described?

Are the findings and conclusions impressive enough to warrant trying them in my practice?

Are there any organizational, logistical, cost, or time barriers to incorporating this approach into my practice? Could they be overcome?

What changes, additions, training, or purchases would be needed to start using this approach?

SHOULD I CHANGE MY PRACTICE BASED ON THESE FINDINGS? Yes _____ No _____

Once I change my practice, how will I know if the change has improved the care I give?

Appraisal of the Evidence From a Research-Based Practice Guideline

---

Citation

Synopsis

What does the guideline address?
What population of patients is the guideline intended for?
What are the key decision points addressed by the guideline?
What outcomes are addressed by the guideline?
What process was used to develop the guideline?

Credibility Profile

Are the guidelines based on a comprehensive meta-analysis or integrative research review?
Is the scientific basis for each recommendation provided?
Are all the key decision points addressed?
At each decision point, was the full range of actions evaluated?
Does the discussion of the way the panel reached decisions convince us that all evidence was considered in an impartial manner?
Are the guidelines current?
Was the panel that developed the guideline made up of people with the necessary skills, expertise, and backgrounds?

ARE THE RECOMMENDATIONS CREDIBLE? Yes _____ No _____

Applicability Profile

Does the guideline address a problem, decision, or situation we see in our practice?
Would we be using all or just part of the guideline? Specify what parts.
Are the recommended courses of action acceptable and feasible to us and our patients?
To follow the guideline, what will we have to do differently?
Do we have the resources, skills, and equipment to implement this guideline accurately and safely?

SHOULD WE ADOPT THIS GUIDELINE IN ITS ENTIRETY? Yes _____ No _____

Should we adopt parts of it? _____
What will we have to do to implement the change?
How will we know if our patients are benefiting from our use of the guideline?

Glossary

Accuracy A term used to characterize a physiologic or physical measurement instrument; it is the ability of the instrument to (a) identify correctly the signal of interest, (b) produce a positive test in persons who have the condition or state, and (c) produce a negative test in persons who do not have the condition or state.

Applicability judgment The appraiser's overall judgment regarding whether a finding is likely to transfer well to a particular population or setting; the issues of whether the same outcomes are likely to be realized and whether the practitioner will be able to safely and effectively use the innovation based on the finding are the major considerations of the applicability judgment.

Appraisal The evaluative estimation of the scientific credibility, clinical significance, and applicability of research evidence.

Case-control study A retrospective, quasi-experimental study in which cases are identified after an outcome of interest has occurred and compared to a control group who did not experience the outcome; the comparison looks backward using records and interviews to discover antecedent factors that may have contributed to the different outcomes of the two groups.

Clinical question A question relevant to clinical practice for which a practitioner seeks research evidence as a source of knowledge.

Clinical significance An appraiser's judgment that a particular research finding is large enough to make a practical, clinical difference in patients' well-being or outcomes.

Cohort study A prospective, quasi-experimental study in which groups with and without an exposure or treatment are formed in a nonrandom manner and followed over time with respect to clinical outcomes.

Collective evidence Findings from two or more studies relevant to a particular topic or clinical question.

Composition of evidence The make-up of the evidence; some evidence is made up of findings that all address the same aspect of an issue, whereas other evidence is made up of findings addressing different aspects of an issue.

Conceptual map A thinking tool that helps one see the relationships among variables in a complex situation. It is a diagram of all variables that influence a particular outcome with lines showing associations among the variables.

Confidence interval The range of score values around a point estimate within which the population parameter is likely to lie; the point estimate and confidence interval are based on data from a single or a pooled sample.

Consistent evidence A situation in which findings from two or more studies all point in the same direction or a preponderance of them point in the same direction (moderately consistent evidence).

243

Construct validity A characteristic of a measuring instrument or rating tool describing the extent to which the instrument faithfully portrays the state or attribute it represents, and not some other state or attribute.

Credibility The overall judgment that a particular finding is believable, meaning that the finding faithfully and accurately portrays a real-world event, process, cause-and-effect relationship, or experience. Believability rests on the scientific soundness of the research methods, particularly the control of extraneous variables.

Database A computerized or print compilation of published references/documents with a certain focus, e.g., nursing and allied health, medicine, cancer, or psychology.

Dichotomous data Data characterized by one of two categories, e.g., improvement/no improvement, return to work/no return to work.

Effect size The size of the impact one variable has on another variable, most often the size of impact a treatment variable has on an outcome variable. Several statistics and measures are used to portray the size of this impact in standardized numerical terms.

End-point outcome Patient health event, experience, behavior, activity, or permanent condition that contributes to patient's daily life experiences. Examples of end-point outcomes are: return to work/no return to work, comfort/discomfort, successful coping/failure to cope, frequent/infrequent/no ear infections during a certain time frame, presence/absence of falls, occurrence/non-occurrence of a disease-related event (e.g., amputation), quality of life, performance of a self-care activity.

Evaluation of research-based innovation The collection and analysis of data within a practice setting or organization for the purpose of determining whether a research-based innovation has achieved the benefits that were anticipated.

Evidence-based medicine The integration of individual clinical expertise with the best available evidence from systematic research (Sackett et al., 1997).

False negative findings Results that are interpreted as meaning that there is not a statistically significant difference between the outcomes of the groups compared or a statistically significant association among variables, when in reality there was a difference that the study design and analysis failed to detect.

False positive findings Results that are interpreted as meaning that there is a statistically significant difference between the outcomes of the groups compared or a statistically significant association among variables, when in reality there was no difference.

Inconsistent evidence Evidence from two or more studies that is variable or contradictory, meaning that the findings of the studies were not all in the same direction or were of different magnitude.

Incremental usage A way of using research findings whereby the practitioner changes a particular action or adds an element to how something is done but does not adopt a whole new approach to doing it.

Integrative research review (also called qualitative synthesis)   Analysis and synthesis of data from two or more studies using summation, logical synthesis, and narrative characterization.

Intermediate outcome   An indicator of a patient health state, capability, risk, or evolving condition that is thought to lead to a particular end-point outcome although not always in a direct manner or time frame. Examples of intermediate outcomes are: a clinical laboratory value, stress test result, score on an anxiety scale, perceived self-efficacy, intention to enact a health behavior, risk for falling, myocardial perfusion.

Internal validity   The degree to which it can be inferred that the effects that were observed in a study are the results of the independent variable rather than uncontrolled extraneous factors.

Measures of clinical significance   Numerical portrayal of findings that gives them clinical meaning. The most commonly used measures are absolute risk reduction, relative risk, relative risk reduction, numbers needed to treat, and difference in means. These measures aid the appraiser in reaching a judgment about the clinical significance of a particular finding.

Meta-analysis   (also called quantitative synthesis) Analysis and synthesis of data from two or more studies using statistical techniques to combine results across studies.

Pathways of research-based practice   Three distinct courses of action within research-based practice; these pathways involve appraisal of (a) state-of-the-science summaries, (b) collective evidence from two or more studies, and (c) findings from a single research study.

Point estimate   The best estimate of an unknown population value; it is based on the data from a single sample or on the pooled results from several samples.

Precision   A term used to characterize a physiologic or physical measurement instrument; it is the ability of the instrument to reliably detect small change (or fine variation) in the condition or state of interest.

r^2 (coefficient of determination)   This statistic portrays the amount of shared influence between two variables, meaning the amount of variance in each that results from its relationship with the other.

Random assignment (also called randomization)   A procedure used to assign individual participants in a study to a treatment or control group in a manner whereby each participant has an equal chance of being assigned to either group.

Reducing the set   Steps taken by a practitioner to limit the number of studies that need to be appraised to answer the clinical question; the limiting should be done in a way that avoids bias and includes studies most relevant to the clinical question.

Reliability   The degree of consistency with which an instrument measures the attribute it was designed to measure.

Research design   The blueprint for conducting a study, including purpose, methods of collecting and analyzing data, and specification of how the quality of the data will be assured and extraneous variables will be controlled.

Research evidence   Knowledge produced by conducting a research study or by summarizing research findings from two or more studies; the three main forms of research evidence are findings from a single study, collective findings from two or more studies, and state-of-the-science summaries.

Research utilization   The process by which scientifically produced knowledge is transferred to practice.

Research-based practice   The considered used of research findings and collective research evidence by health care practitioners to guide approaches to care, specific courses of action, and recommendations made to individual patients.

Research-based practice guidelines   (also called research-based clinical guidelines) Specific recommendations regarding the care of a particular patient population that are based on a review of the research relative to the various decision points involved in the care.

Research-practice gap   A knowledge situation in which knowledge relevant to practice has been produced using research, but a long time passes between the time the finding is produced and when it is widely incorporated into practice.

Sensitivity   The true positive rate of an instrument's measurements; the likelihood that a person with the attribute will have a positive test result using the instrument.

Soft usage   A way of using research findings whereby the practitioner allows a finding to influence his or her understanding or thinking about a certain kind of situation without a specific plan to change practice.

Specificity   The true negative rate of an instrument's measurements; the likelihood that a person without the attribute will have a negative test result using the instrument.

State-of-the-science summary   Several forms of research evidence involving the collective evidence of results or findings from more than one study are analyzed together to produce an overall finding or conclusion regarding the body of evidence. The three forms of state-of-the-science summaries are meta-analysis, integrative research reviews, and research-based practice guidelines.

Statistical significance   A term indicating the likelihood that the results of a study may have occurred by chance is less than a specified level of probability.

Strong evidence   Evidence from two or more credible studies that is consistent across studies, and was produced by studies using the types of design that best answer the research question.

Substantial change   A way of using research findings in practice whereby the practitioner makes a major change in how something is done.

Sufficiency of evidence   The completeness of the evidence about a topic, issue, or relationship among variables.

Synopsis A concise statement of the essential elements of a study, i.e., purpose, methods, findings.

Telnet A computer-to-computer connection via telephone lines. A frequent application in research-based practice is to call another library and search their catalog just as if you were using the computer in that library.

Theory-in-use The everyday, explanatory understanding a practitioner uses to informally organize her thinking about a certain kind of clinical situation. The term was originated by Schon (1983).

References

Sackett, D.L., Richardson, W.S., Rosenberg, W., and Haynes, R.B. (1997). *Evidence-Based Medicine: How to Practice and Teach EBM.* New York: Churchill Livingstone.

Schon, D.A. (1983). *The Reflective Practitioner: How Professionals Think in Action.* New York: Basic Books.

Index